THE
TAMING
of the
CHEW

For Sally—
Remember to
make self-loving
Choices—

♡
Denise Lamothe

9/21/99

What people are saying about

The Taming of the Chew . . .

"Finally a book which views psychological and physiological dependencies on a number of levels. It combines practical holistic knowledge with compassion and common sense. Not only fast and easy reading but *The Taming of the Chew* is a valuable resource for all of us!"

Joan L. Day, MS in Natural Health

"At last a book that makes sense. *The Taming of the Chew* is a sensible, refreshing, comprehensive book that not only explains compulsive eating behavior but also is filled with practical, realistic ways to manage this problem. It is clear to me that Denise Lamothe really cares. I'll be keeping her book at my bedside at all times and referring to it often."

Amy Rae Perez

"I did not realize the depth of obsession experienced by my patients with eating disorders. This insightful presentation has made me more aware and hopefully more effective as a health care provider."

Laurie Kelleher, Physician Assistant

"My eyes have been opened to the overwhelming issue of food obsession. I have learned much about self-care techniques and personal "response-ability" which will be helpful in my work with clients as a massage therapist. Denise Lamothe presents this valuable information with much insight, compassion, warmth and practicality. Her willingness to share her personal experiences enhances the material presented. A consciousness-raising work well worth reading!"

Sharon A. Piantedosi, RN, CLMT
(certified licensed massage therapist)

"Denise Lamothe has succeeded in integrating many divergent theoretical perspectives into a coherent philosophy and method for overcoming overeating. Humanistic Psychology, Self-in-Relation Theory, Cognitive-Behavioral techniques, addictions theory, Holistic Medicine, and spirituality are skillfully interwoven with poignant personal accounts of her clients' and her own experiences with overeating and recovery. She has created a thoughtful plan for regaining control over food. This is a very personal book: Readers, both overeaters and therapists, will find words of wisdom and ideas for action within it. I will definitely be recommending it to my clients."

Marc Wilson, Ph.D.
NH Certified Psychologist, Eating Disorders Specialist

"Denise Lamothe's *The Taming of the Chew* looks at compulsive overeating in an open honest manner. Although geared towards a female audience, the book can easily apply to men who also struggle to *"Tame the Chew."* This book is useful for both lay persons and trained professionals and I have chosen it as suggested reading for the students in my Addictive Disorders class."

Wayne K. Cunningham, RN,MA,LADC

"This book goes way beyond common knowledge. It covers compulsive eating issues in a truly holistic way, offering helpful suggestions to manage eating problems on physical, emotional, social and spiritual levels. It is amazingly comprehensive and validating and is valuable resource for anyone—practitioners, clients and educators alike. I highly recommend it!"

Mimi L. Smith, LMSW

"*The Taming of the Chew* is an easily read book full of marvelous, practical ideas in which Denise Lamothe combines much insight, experience and research. The focus is not only on eating issues but also on learning to love yourself. Only when you have learned this will your *Chew be Tamed.*"

Jane Bunker, RNC

THE

TAMING

of the

CHEW

A Holistic Guide to Stopping Compulsive Eating

By Denise Lamothe, Psy.D., H.H.D.

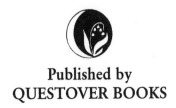

Published by
QUESTOVER BOOKS

Questover Books
PO Box 933
Epping, New Hampshire 03042

E-Mail: QUESTDCL@aol.com
Web site: http://www.questover.com

Telephone/FAX: (603) 679-2432

Printed in the United States of America
First Printing: June 1998

ISBN 0-9663653-0-5

Illustration by Sean Hopkins, Manchester, New Hampshire
Photo by Philip Scalia, Exeter, New Hampshire

Dedicated with pride, love and
respect to my friend and teacher—
my daughter, Mimi.

*A*cknowledgments

A S with any project, a book is the creation of many. This work is no exception. It comes to you through the efforts and generosity of many people and I could not have produced it without each of them. My deepest thanks to:

...my friend, Eric Mart, whose humor and encouragement helped me muster the courage I needed to begin.

...Laurie Blakeney, my editor, consultant, and friend, for her guidance and personal interest.

...Betsy Arnold, Sharon Piantedosi, Laurie Kelleher, Joan Day, Mimi Hopkins, Marc Wilson, Amy Perez, Jane Bunker, Sharon Lupien, Lisa Hoffman and Wayne Cunningham, who enthusiastically agreed to read my work or listen to my audiotapes and who sensitively delivered the feedback necessary for completion of this work.

...Patricia Maher for her invaluable assistance with cover design and creation.

...Jack Beckwith for sheparding me through the final stages of this project.

...my children, Sean, Mimi and Shane Hopkins for helping me to maintain my sense of humor and to Sean for technical assistance and for patiently answering all my computer questions without laughing.

...my brother, Paul Lamothe, and sister-in-law, Tobie, for the use of their retirement home where I was able to seclude myself and find the peace and quiet I needed.

...my partner, Betsy Arnold for helping with the cover design, donating hours of her time to give me computer assistance and for her unfailing patience, love and support. I thank her for being amazingly clear and for nurturing me whenever I became discouraged and frustrated along the way. Mostly I thank her for always being there and believing in me.

...my five grandchildren for reminding me so often of what is truly important in this lifetime—loving, having fun, being in the present, and keeping things in perspective.

Most of all, I am indebted to the hundreds of women who have entered my office through the years and trusted me with the most intimate details of their painful and courageous lives. Thanks to each of you for helping me to learn and grow with you. You have been my greatest teachers.

Without all of these remarkably special people there would be no book to write, no story to tell.

About the Author

DENISE LAMOTHE is a New Hampshire Certified Psychologist and a Doctor of Holistic Health. She earned her Masters Degree in Counseling Psychology in 1981, and her Doctorate in Clinical Psychology in 1989, from Antioch/New England Graduate School in Keene, New Hampshire, and her Doctorate in Holistic Health in 1997 from The Clayton School of Natural Healing in Birmingham, Alabama. Dr. Lamothe has worked with a variety of populations over time including emotionally disturbed adolescents, children and adults. She spent several years working at The Stone Center at Wellesley College in Wellesley, Massachusetts providing counseling, consultation and education to the campus community. While working there with Jean Baker Miller, M.D., and colleagues, Dr. Lamothe studied Self-in-Relation Theory, a theory of women's development which originated at The Stone Center and greatly informs her work today. She completed her post doctoral training at Lake Shore Hospital in Manchester, New Hampshire as a Staff Psychologist on the Child and Adolescent unit and was instrumental in establishing a unit exclusively for women based on the Stone Center model.

Dr. Lamothe has taught for The N. H. Technical Institute, New England College and Antioch/New England Graduate School and has provided consultation and education to a variety of agencies including N.H. Partners in Education, The Visiting Nurse's Association, Manchester City Library, Appletree Education, The Multiple Sclerosis Society, The Massachusetts Holistic Nursing Association and Notre Dame College. She is a member of the N.H. Psychological Association, The American Psychological Association, The Association for Women in Psychology and the American Naturopathic Medical Association.

Dr. Lamothe has been in private practice since 1981. She combines traditional and alternative methods to work "holistically"— that is, with each client's physical, emotional and spiritual needs. Special areas of expertise include eating disorders, life transitions, midlife and menopause, alternative lifestyles, anxiety, depression and stress. She has helped people with compulsive eating behaviors since she opened her practice and runs weekend retreats and workshops for people who struggle with this issue. Currently Dr. Lamothe resides in Epping, New Hampshire and is in private practice there.

Contents

Introduction

AS reported in *Modern Maturity* magazine (May-June 1998) "With the exception of the population of a few Pacific islands, Americans are the fattest people on earth." Why are so many of us overweight? Why are so many of us prone to eating to excess? Why are we obsessed with food and body size? For many of us, food has long been a source of anxiety. Alternating between *eating compulsively* for periods of time and then *dieting* for a while has been our life-long style of food "management." This pattern is self-destructive and leads to obesity, high blood pressure, low self-esteem, depression, anxiety, a general sense of being out of control and other problems. We are all different but most women suffer at least occasionally with food issues. For many of us, food control has seemed impossible at times. And, for some of us, compulsive eating has become a life-style.

Because you have chosen to purchase and read this book, I am assuming you eat more than you wish to eat at least occasionally (or you know someone who does). Some of you may binge-eat infrequently and some more often. The behavior of overindulging is common and nearly everyone eats more than they need or want to at times. Because you feel out of control with food sometimes does not necessarily mean a pathological condition exists.

Following is a clinical description of a "binge eater" which I have excerpted from *The Diagnostic and Statistical Manual of Mental Disorders Fourth Edition* (DSM IV, 1994) used by the American Psychiatric and Psychological Associations to identify and diagnose various disorders. One condition that they have labeled "binge-eating disorder" pertains to persons who eat in an out of control way. Following is a list of criteria that must be met in order for this diagnosis to apply. Please read the following information carefully. If you fit the criteria for binge-eating disorder (or if you struggle with

1

Anorexia Nervosa or Bulimia Nervosa), I urge you to consult professionals who are knowledgeable and skilled in the treatment of food control issues.

Binge Eating Disorder

A. Recurrent episodes of binge eating. An episode is characterized by both of the following:
   1. eating, in a discrete period of time (e.g., within any 2-hour period), an amount of food that is definitely larger than most people would eat in a similar period of time under similar circumstances.
   2. a sense of lack of control over eating during the episode (e.g., a feeling that one cannot stop eating or control what or how much one is eating).
B. The binge-eating episodes are associated with three (or more) of the following:
   1. eating much more rapidly than normal
   2. eating until feeling uncomfortably full
   3. eating large amounts of food when not feeling physically hungry
   4. eating alone because of being embarrassed by how much one is eating
   5. feeling disgusted with oneself, depressed, or very guilty after overeating
C. Marked distress regarding binge eating is present.
D. The binge occurs, on average, at least two days a week for six months.
E. The binge eating is not associated with regular use of inappropriate compensatory behaviors (e.g., purging, fasting, excessive exercise) and does not occur exclusively during the course of Anorexia Nervosa or Bulimia Nervosa. (If you are using these inappropriate, dangerous compensatory behaviors please do seek professional help.)

If you did meet the above criteria, begin by scheduling an appointment with your medical doctor for a complete physical (which includes appropriate blood work). You may also wish to consult someone who is open to holistic health and uses alternative practices in his or her work (such as herbal therapy, homeopathy, naturopathy, etc.) You may also want to consult with a nutritionist who is open to alternative eating styles and possibly to meet with a psychologist or psychotherapist. Having this support and guidance can help you use the suggestions in this book effectively. Also, for many of us, it may be useful to view food abuse as a powerful addiction—as a dependency and to locate a professional who can work with us from that perspective. Only you know how problematic food is for you and only you can evaluate the degree to which you are dependent upon food and whether or not you should seek professional help. The information in these pages will be helpful to you whether your intention is to work on this issue by yourself or with a professional. This book will teach you about compulsive eating and will outline ways to stop that behavior.

First, I will share my perspective about compulsive eating behavior and my philosophy of treatment. Please note that our physical bodies and our emotional and spiritual selves are intertwined and that we have been heavily influenced in our society to look and act in certain ways to be accepted and approved of. So, to feel in control of our impulses to eat compulsively, we need to address all of these areas and to map out strategies to bring each of these aspects of ourselves into balance. This requires us to know ourselves physically, emotionally and spiritually and to understand the impact social forces have had on us throughout our lives. This is no small task but it is possible and worthwhile. This book will help you to accomplish this, and to make *your* Individual Plan to stop feeling out of control and eating compulsively.

I have written this book, from both my personal and professional points of view, after having waged my own private war with compulsive eating and dieting—enduring phases of obesity, bulimia and anorexia—having finally found a path to a healthier life with a more positive, balanced and appreciative attitude towards myself, my own body and food. My body is not and will never be "perfect" according to our contemporary societal standard. However, after more than fifty years of walking around on this planet alternately starving and stuffing myself, the idea of perfection has become irrelevant. It has been replaced instead by a feeling of peace and an appreciation of myself and of the many wonderful things my body can do.

This book is not about being thin. It is about loving yourself just the way you are and eating in ways that feel nurturing—not compulsive and self-abusive. You will lose weight if you implement some of the suggestions on the following pages. If you wish to do so, that is fine—but helping you to lose weight is not my primary goal. My wish is to help you to feel healthy, peaceful and happy with yourself regardless of how many pounds you weigh. Please realize that many factors determine our body size—genetic make-up, metabolism, age, etc. We have no control over these, yet many of us have tried to force our bodies to be different than they are able to be. This is not only frustrating, it is futile. Please suspend any plans to mold yourself into a cultural ideal and instead read through these pages with a desire to learn about yourself and to cultivate self-acceptance and self-love in the process. This will help you *Tame Your Chew.*

I have spent countless hours in my role as a therapist listening to my clients' painful histories and experiences and helping them in their personal struggles to control their eating. For nearly twenty years, people have come to share their stories of guilt, self-hatred, shame and frustration. In their pasts, some have lost weight, some have not. Some have developed an ability to accept themselves no matter what their weight may be, and others have abandoned hope, finding the battle against compulsive eating too demanding and discouraging.

This is easy to understand. As I mentioned earlier, the *only* way to overcome feeling out of control and helpless around food is to first understand the issue "holistically." This means to cultivate knowledge and understanding of compulsive eating from many perspectives—considering mind, body and spirit as well as societal factors. We may never completely eliminate urges to eat compulsively. They may manifest from time to time just because we are human beings with appetites. We can, however, learn ways to deal with our urges when they surface and to choose other ways to deal with these compulsions. To do this successfully it is *essential* to understand ourselves in this way. This means to know ourselves physically, mentally and spiritually and to understand the impact that societal messages have had on us. When we pay attention to these aspects of ourselves and view ourselves in this context, we discover ways we have become out of balance. This self-exploration is necessary to achieve balance in all areas of our lives. For example, if we attempt to eat a healthy diet but we ignore other important needs (e.g. our need for exercise, rest, laughter, relationships, attention to our feelings, solitude) we soon find ourselves turning to food as we have in the past—*to fill our needs.* Food, of course, does not fulfill our *real* needs.

We will be forever turning to food to nurture and satisfy ourselves if we don't identify what our *real* needs are and discover ways to fulfill them satisfactorily. I cannot emphasize strongly enough that to do this, we *must* attend to our physical, emotional and spiritual selves. We must also appreciate how we have been shaped by society. This is the context in which our self-destructive behaviors have been encouraged and have flourished.

As a psychologist concerned with helping people overcome the distress of compulsive eating behavior, I have repeatedly witnessed the results of people going from one "helper" to another, finding little or no relief. A psychologist or social worker may offer them some form of therapy—behavioral, cognitive, insight-oriented, etc. A physician or psychiatrist might suggest a medication regime and a nutritionist could contribute strategies for improving diet. A religious or spiritual counselor may offer prayer and spiritual guidance. The staff at a health club could devise an exercise program to help eliminate fat and tone muscle. Many self-help books and tapes contribute knowledge of one or two aspects of compulsive eating behavior. Friends and families may lend their support to the dieter's cause.

In order to overcome the painful compulsion of overeating, you need all accessible, relevant information and a way to make sense of it. This book will help you to do that as it addresses the issue of compulsive eating holistically, in its entirety. Initially, looking at the complete picture may seem too rigorous an undertaking. Some clients have come to me hoping that I would provide a magic answer or a quick solution and, when it became apparent that I had no magic wand or instant "cure," they left to continue their search for someone or something outside of themselves to "fix" them. This book is for people who have tried all the "quick" weight loss diets and gimmicks and have come to realize that they must do something quite different. This book is for you because you are ready to educate yourself and to understand your life experiences and behaviors. It will be a valuable resource because you are ready to begin making these important changes. Greater health and inner peace will be the result of your effort.

I urge you to approach the task of "working" this book with an attitude of openness and play and to be gentle with yourself as you gain insights and experiment with changes. It requires courage to change and to grow and it takes time to evolve—as through any growth process or metamorphosis. By reading this book, educating yourself, and then using the included suggestions as you wish, you can change your course from negative and self-destructive to positive, self-loving and rewarding. Remember, this is not about achieving some societal image of perfection. It is about feeling happier and more relaxed in your body. It is about loving and nurturing yourself. It is about being the happiest and most personally fulfilled you can possibly be.

At first glance, it may seem overwhelming to look at the issue of compulsive eating in so many different ways. However, taking it in one step at a time, one page at a time, will bring the clarity and new levels of understanding that you need to make permanent changes. For each of us the journey towards health and self-appreciation may seem discouraging at times, and its demands too great. Remember that no one is perfect and no one can do everything perfectly. It is instead our task to experiment, to try new behaviors on for size, keep what fits and discard that which does not. In this way each of us makes room to try even more new behaviors. Through this process of experimentation we evolve into healthier, happier beings. Giving ourselves permission to grow and change, to play, to adjust and readjust our attitudes and behaviors redefines our life as a creative, rewarding adventure. This has proven true for me and for nearly all of the clients I have counseled. It also can and will for you.

In Part I, I will share information to help you understand food control issues from the four perspectives we have discussed: physically, emotionally, socially and spiritually. As you explore these perspectives, you will develop a greater understanding of what your personal behavior is all about. The complex issue of food abusive behavior will become more understandable and clear. The de-mystifying of your process will help you to feel less anxious and fearful around food and you will gradually cultivate the ability to think your actions through *before* overeating. Then you will be able to make responsible, healthy, self-loving choices more often.

In Part II, I will share many suggestions and exercises to help you in your healing process. Again, I will divide the issue into the four perspectives and consider changes you may make to heal *holistically*. I will share my own experiences where I think they may be helpful and draw upon the wisdom of the many clients I have worked with, sharing their stories while of course guarding individual identities. In Part III, I will help you make an individual plan for yourself and you will have the opportunity to think about how to care for your body's needs in a loving, healthful way. This process will be different for each of you. There is no "right" way to do it. You will be encouraged to pay attention to your own inner voice of wisdom and to forge your own unique path to a healthy, rewarding way of life.

At the end of each Chapter, you will find a page entitled "Reflections." Use this space to make notes, draw pictures or scribble on. Taking a few minutes to pause and reflect before you continue will help you to absorb what you are reading and will give you a chance to note points that have been especially relevant to your experience. Use these pages to capture your thoughts and feelings at that moment and reflect on them. Then move on.

Following these sections you will find a list of useful concepts to remember. Reviewing these regularly is helpful and will enable you to keep the knowledge you have gained fresh in your mind. This will help you prevent relapsing into old, self-destructive, compulsive behaviors. In addition to this, you will find a reading list at the back of the book that contains references for books I have referred to in the text as well as many others that I think you will find useful. These can help you increase your knowledge in any of the areas we will touch upon—physical, emotional, social and spiritual. Finally, you will discover a list of resources which you will find helpful.

Think of the reasons you initially picked this book up. What motivated you? What were you hoping to find within these pages? I hope you will share this goal with me: that, by "working" this book, exploring your personal journey and learning to deeply understand yourself, you will be able to create a plan for taking the best possible care of yourself—a plan designed by you and for you which exactly fits your special needs. This plan will help you fulfill your commitment to eliminate long-standing, self-destructive behaviors—to *Tame your Chew.*

This book will not have all the answers. It is not meant to be another leg of a discouraging journey. It is, instead, intended to help you start on an exciting journey towards inner peace and self-love. It is my hope that as you read this book you will begin to generate ideas that work specifically for you. I will help you to do this by giving you tools you may use to construct your personal long-range plan. Please join me on this quest with an attitude of curiosity and exploration. Be gentle with yourself. Put aside any expectations about your weight for the moment and relax. The information you are about to absorb will help you to understand yourself and your behaviors. It will demystify the painful issue of compulsive eating and help you feel better about yourself and your body. *Adopting an attitude of curiosity, exploration, self-discovery and self-love (now and from this moment on) empowers you to make the changes necessary to achieve and maintain balance in all areas of your life. This will help you arrive at a natural and comfortable weight and to finally quiet the insistent, destructive tantrums of your Chew.*

What Is the Chew?

WHAT is the Chew? The Chew is our saboteur. She is a devious, powerful, destructive little creature who is always lurking somewhere within us to sabotage our most sincere and ambitious attempts to stop eating compulsively. The Chew is not a stranger to the millions of us who have struggled with food control issues for a lifetime. She is a ravenous, despicable monster who lures us into donut shops and candy stores and who crams food into our mouths with brute force. She is a hurtful, persistent, out of control part of each of us. As you read the following pages you will become well acquainted with your personal Chew and you will learn ways to cope with her. By the conclusion of this book you will be intimately familiar with your Chew and you will be fully equipped to win your battles against compulsive eating.

Please approach this experience in an open way. Suspend any expectations you now hold about your eating behavior. It has taken you years to become a compulsive eater. Your Chew has been in charge for a long time and it will take a bit of time to reverse old, self-destructive behaviors. Be patient and gentle with yourself as you learn about your personal Chew and you will discover ways to neutralize her power. As you become more familiar with her you will be able to sense her presence before she has you in her tenacious grasp. You will be able to maintain control over yourself, your eating behavior and your life.

You can never be free of your Chew entirely. She has been with you since your earliest years and she is a vital part of your humanness. You can, however, learn to accept her as part of you and to ignore her destructive mandates. You can *Tame your Chew*. You *can* live free from insistent urges to binge. This book will teach you how.

PART I

UNDERSTANDING THE ISSUES—
WHAT'S GOING ON?

FOOD abusive behavior is about a lot of things. It is about how we are feeling about ourselves at the moment, about self-love and self-hatred. It's about feeling out of balance and disconnected. It's also about what's going on in our bodies on a cellular level and about how tired or how stressed we feel. Food abuse has to do with the quality of our relationships and the environment in which we live. It has to do with what our hormones are up to and what season it is of the year. Destructive and/or healthy food behaviors tie in with our attitudes about ourselves and others and the world in which we live; and with the messages we have carried with us from the time we were children. What we eat, where, when, how and with whom we eat, are all important pieces of information for us to explore if we are to serve our bodies well and manage our own needs effectively. Selecting what we put into our bodies and the ways that we manage that process are complex phenomena to say the least. Urges to eat are amazingly strong and we can easily feel overpowered by them. We may sometimes feel that we have no say in the matter at all. Urges overwhelm us. We feel helpless to stop or control them.

Does the following scenario sound familiar? You notice you are hungry. This may be actual physical hunger but, most likely, it is not. It is probably *emotional* hunger of some sort. Perhaps you are feeling lonely, or afraid, or depleted, or angry. Whatever the reason, the urge to put something into your mouth builds in intensity. You decide to have a little something to "take the edge off." Maybe a small salad or a rice cake with a little peanut butter on it. You eat that but do not feel satisfied. You may feel even hungrier than when you began. So you decide to eat a bit more, believing that food is what you need to satisfy your hunger (although it is not).

You remember those cookies that were left over from the party three days ago. You're off to the pantry in a flash. As the cookies disappear into your mouth, you remember the gallon of ice cream sitting and waiting for you in the freezer. You bought it for guests next Friday night, but you know you have time to replace it before then. Before the cookies have had a chance to arrive in your stomach, your spoon is deep into the ice cream and your other hand is reaching for that jar of fudge sauce you keep for "emergencies." You have, at that point, crossed what I call the "what-the-hell line."

You no longer think at all. You are on a mission. Anything digestible is fair game. Your physical, emotional and spiritual needs are still not getting met but you continue to cram food down your throat in a vain attempt to soothe yourself. You eat everything in reach, but remain unsatisfied. Your real needs are being ignored and most likely you will end up feeling guilty, ashamed and frustrated. You vow never to eat in an "out of control" way like this again. But the next time always comes. The urges do return and you feel helpless to resist them once again. You feel trapped in this cycle. You want to take care of yourself and, despite all your resolve, you repeat this pattern of wanton eating again and again. Does this seem familiar? How often have you crossed the "what-the-hell line" and blamed yourself after? How often have you felt helpless to stop a binge?

To be successful at managing eating behavior, it is helpful to understand why food intake is so difficult to control. If we have no idea why we are doing something, our chances of changing that behavior are minimal. Instead, we tend to view our behavior as mysterious and beyond our control. If we examine some of the motives behind our out-of-control eating behavior and gain insights into our own personal reasons for overeating, we can demystify the process and empower ourselves to make different, informed choices.

Following is a discussion of some of the more common reasons for overeating. Perhaps you will recognize how some of these relate to your experience. Maybe some will not feel relevant or you will think of reasons not mentioned that will provide you with insights. Remember this book delivers general information. It is up to you to read with discretion and to take in what makes sense for you in your particular life circumstances. The more you can personalize the readings, the more helpful this book will be. Let's begin by taking a quick look at some common reasons for overeating. Later in various sections of the book we will consider each of them in more detail and talk about better ways to deal with them.

CHAPTER I

General Reasons for Overeating

THERE are many reasons for overeating. We eat when we are sad, when we are happy, when we are lonely or tense. We may eat any time and for just about any reason. As anyone who overeats well knows, we need no excuse to abuse ourselves with too much food. It takes no effort. For many of us, the process of stuffing ourselves with food has been automatic. The food goes in with very little thought or notice. My clients sometimes look at this robotic behavior and say, "That's just me. It's just the way I am!" The reality is, however, that it is not "you." It is not "just how you are." You are a person with a certain eye color, certain height, certain skin tone. Thoughtless out-of-control eating is not "you." It is, instead, a behavior that you have learned and *any behavior can be changed.*

Many women who have difficulty controlling their eating behavior report feeling out of control in other areas of their lives as well. Perhaps their relationships are less than satisfying or someone close to them is ill or in emotional pain. As women, we have often viewed ourselves as "soothers" or "givers." We may imagine that it is our innate responsibility to keep all those around us free from any form of pain or suffering. We respond to everyone else's needs and lose sight of our own. We allow others to occupy the spaces in our minds and hearts. We push ourselves out of the picture instead of keeping ourselves and our needs in the foreground. We think we have to protect

15

everyone. It doesn't matter that this is impossible. If, for example, we see a loved one experiencing distress, we may feel guilty and upset —as if we are personally responsible for *their* pain. There are good reasons for this and for the many other distorted perceptions we experience. We will look more closely at why we tend to take responsibility for others in the sections on emotional and social reasons for overeating. *For the moment, just know that feeling out of control with food generally means you are feeling out of control in other areas of your life as well.* Now let's begin by looking at some other common reasons for compulsive eating.

ENMESHED, ABANDONED, OUT OF CONTROL

We eat when we perceive our independence as threatened by others—when people seem too "close." We also eat when others seem too "far away" from us. Because we cannot always control the level of intimacy we experience with another, we feel afraid and out of control. Then we seek food to soothe the anxiety that comes with these feelings. How close or distant to be with another is difficult to know at times. Healthy relationships require a flow—a give and take—of energy. Most of us were never taught how to achieve and maintain appropriate levels of intimacy—how to dance with the changing rhythms in a relationship. This takes knowledge and practice.

You have heard of "dysfunctional families." You will most likely have a personal connotation around that term. Some of us are comfortable with the concept, others of us have strongly negative assumptions about it. The term is used and misused in our culture to explain every form of wellness or illness. For our purpose here, let me define what I consider "dysfunctional families." These are families where the members usually are not able to be genuine and honest with each other. Communication is poor or non-existent and family members can feel either isolated from each other and abandoned—or totally enmeshed in each other's lives and feelings. Either way, the result is the same. We end up confused and feel out of control. We fail to learn what good boundaries are and how to set appropriate limits. No one helps us to understand the feelings we are having or teaches us how to manage these feelings and experiences in a healthy way. We will discuss this in more depth later in the section on psychological reasons for eating behaviors. *For the moment, suffice it to say that one reason a woman may eat in an "out-of-control" way is because she cannot control the experiences and feelings of those around her.*

TRANSITIONS

Another difficult time for many of us to approach our eating behaviors in a thoughtful way is when we find ourselves in any kind of transition. Transition means any time of change—any time when there are important decisions to make or conflicting feelings to experience. We may be moving to a new location, beginning a new job, having a child, graduating from or entering school, for example. It is common to feel fearful and overwhelmed when we face change. Transition also means any movement, growth, or challenge. A woman may be changing her marital status, entering her menopausal years, coping with illness or caring for aging parents or a sick child. Transition can also be as simple as getting in the car to go from one location to another. (Have you ever wondered why you sometimes feel "driven" to binge while you are driving?) *So be aware that whenever you are involved in any process of growth and facing change you may be particularly susceptible to overeating and your Chew may seem particularly powerful at that time.*

MEDICATING FEELINGS

Another common reason to overeat is to anesthetize uncomfortable feelings. Change is a part of life and it is generally accompanied by many feelings. Some may be pleasant, some not, but *all* feelings are valid and necessary. If we pay attention to our cravings and urges to eat we can use our experiences with food as barometers that give us valuable information about our feelings. For example if we crave crunchy foods that allow us to use our jaws powerfully, we might be angry. If we seek creamy, soothing foods, such as ice cream or puddings, we might be lonely or sad and seeking consolation.

If we notice what we are feeling and then pay attention to these feelings they will give us valuable information about the choices we are making and the experiences we are having. Often, however, we fail to pay attention to these urges and act on them instead. When we fail to attend to our feelings and deny or suppress them instead we set ourselves up to binge. Food provides a way of medicating ourselves so we will *not feel* difficult feelings and many of us learned how effective this is long ago. If we feel anxious, tense, depressed, bored or scared, for example, we might head for the kitchen to sedate ourselves with sugars, fats and carbohydrates. If we feel angry, we might stuff ourselves to keep a lid on things. This often works in the short term but, in the long run, we still have to deal with the situations that provoked these feelings. The longer we wait to deal with difficult situations, the harder they are to confront.

Our feelings are to be honored and valued—not numbed with food or other substances. Later, when we examine ways to heal in Part II, we will discuss some healthier ways to cope with life situations and to deal with distressing feelings. There are other ways—ways that are far more effective and satisfying. *For the moment, it is enough just to realize that our feelings are interwoven with our eating behaviors and that we don't need to use food to manage our feelings.*

CELEBRATING AND SOCIALIZING

Have you ever paid attention to how focused our culture is on food? Virtually every occasion we experience has food as a central theme. Think of Thanksgiving without turkey and pumpkin pie or Easter without candy eggs. How about Valentine's Day with no chocolate, birthdays or weddings with no cake or even meetings without refreshment breaks? How often do we get together with friends without including food? We ask people to meet us for breakfast, brunch, lunch or dinner. We invite them over for coffee or a drink. When was the last time someone asked you to get together just to spend time enjoying each other's company? Food is everywhere and a part of nearly every occasion.

How can we take care of ourselves in this food-oriented culture? How can we socialize with friends, celebrate birthdays, go to fine restaurants and relax about it? How can we manage to enjoy ourselves, eat only some of what is offered and feel satisfied? How can we survive this constant exposure to food? If we eat too much, the result is anxiety and we will want to eat to medicate this feeling. If we eat too little, we feel deprived and set ourselves up to binge later. If we have weight to lose, we feel anxious about that and if we have lost the weight we wanted to lose, we feel anxious that we will gain it back. (Many women report that they find it much harder to maintain weight loss than to lose the weight in the first place.) So we eat because we *have not* lost weight and we eat because we *have* lost weight. What a dilemma! At either end of the scale, anxiety lurks and if we don't know healthy ways to cope with the anxiety, we eat.

It is impossible to be harmonious, balanced and content all the time in social situations or in life in general. If we feel too successful or unsuccessful, for example, we find ourselves off balance and anxious. Anytime things are a little too "good" or a little too "bad" we find ourselves racing to the refrigerator in search of something to help us find emotional balance. We mistakenly think food can provide this for us. It can not. Only we have the power to cope with our own difficult feelings as we negotiate our way along our own life's path.

All this can be very confusing and discouraging. We will talk about ways to keep our needs in the foreground and to nurture ourselves in Part II. Even in settings where opportunities to sabotage ourselves abound and our Chew is screaming for "treats," we do not have to feel helpless and victimized. *It may be hard for you to believe at this point, but it is possible to feel under control even in the most food-focused situations.*

REWARD AND PUNISHMENT

We both reward and punish ourselves with food because as children we were most likely rewarded and punished with food. In my home, for example, desserts were withheld until all of the vegetables had disappeared. We were given cookies or candy for reinforcement if we behaved and, if we were "extra good," we could have popcorn or a snack late in the evening. You may have been sent to bed without supper as a punishment or not allowed the ice cream or candy others received because you had been "bad." For most, if not all of us, there are memories of food being used in these ways. Food is a powerful motivator. Behavior modification programs use candies, for example, to change difficult behaviors in children or in people who are learning impaired. Once the child or adult learns that he or she will receive a candy when they perform a specific behavior, they become motivated to perform that behavior again to receive another treat. It is extremely effective.

We have all been conditioned in this same way to some extent. If we learned as children that food is a reward, we may continue to use

> My "Onion" Punishment!

it in that way and the deprivation we experience on any diet plan may translate to us as punishment. If food was withheld from us when we were little to keep us in line, we may feel angry now when we experience any hunger. We may rebel against those who punished us then by eating even more now than we really want or need. Begin to notice how often you give yourself a "treat" as a reward. Notice how often you feel deprived and punished at times when you are restricting food.

Taking responsibility for what we put into our mouths means, in part, releasing some of our old beliefs about food. If we can appreciate food as neutral—not good or bad—we can begin making more thoughtful choices. Food is a powerful force in each of our lives. It is hard to untangle our present eating behaviors from the ways we viewed and experienced eating in our childhood years. It is helpful to recognize this and to begin paying attention to the ways you may be using food to reward yourself or how you may be experiencing even mild hunger as a punishment. *If you realize your tendencies to do this, you will be less compelled to act on impulse and you can give yourself time to decide whether you really want to eat or not.*

THE ILLUSION OF ENERGIZING

Food gives us energy and we need the right amount of the right nutrients for our body to function properly. Often, however, we fool ourselves into thinking we need to eat when our body actually does not need more food. For example, when we are tired (i.e. when we need to sleep), we might think we need to eat food to energize our body. Although this may be the case at times, such as in a life or death situation, usually, for compulsive eaters, the food is being used to save us from experiencing our feelings. When we feel tired, angry, frustrated, anxious, bored, lonely, unappreciated or afraid, for example, food becomes a quick and easy way to seemingly perk us up and fill the void we are experiencing. It is easier to tear open a bag of chips or pull a chocolate bar out of the candy machine than it is to sit with those painful feelings.

Feelings of hunger are tricky and often have nothing to do with the fueling of our body. Our body doesn't need excessive amounts of potato chips, chocolate or macaroni and cheese to function optimally, so when we tell ourselves we *need* them for energy, *we are not telling ourselves the truth.* Fats, sugar or caffeine may give us a temporary rush of energy—but this is short-lived, and masking discomfort will leave us feeling even more "tired" than before because we are not giving our body the nutrients it really needs to "energize." So, when we choose sugars, fats or excess carbohydrates we may not be truly, physically hungry. *Cravings we experience deliver valuable messages to us about what we really feel and what we really need.* Our job is to pay attention to these messages and to give ourselves what we really need at the time. Proper rest, a healthful diet, and a peaceful lifestyle give us energy—not junk foods. They may be what our Chew clamors for from time to time, but they are not what we really need.

SECONDARY GAINS

I often ask clients what they are getting out of their compulsive eating behavior. Most look at me as if I'm from another planet and insist that they get absolutely no benefits from eating compulsively or from being overweight. I can understand their surprised reactions, for how can an issue which feels so painful and all-consuming bring with it any *advantages*? Inevitably, when I suggest we talk about the possibility, people resist the idea. "How can this weight or this behavior bring me anything *positive*?" they ask. It seems too hard to think about, impossible to imagine. I often tell them the following story to illustrate my point:

Once I was working with a woman who had been steadily gaining weight since the birth of her first child. She was referred to me by her medical doctor when her weight began seriously taking its toll on her health. She was dangerously obese when we met and was becoming increasingly depressed and discouraged. We worked together for quite a while and, despite all of her best efforts and mine, she continued to put on more weight. Sporadically she would make attempts to take control of her eating but nothing was effective.

One day, after several months of unsuccessful weight loss attempts, we began talking about her family situation and she disclosed to me that her husband badly wanted another child. Her first child, an extremely active little boy, kept her busy constantly and she strongly resisted the idea of adding to their family (and thus her workload). She feared her husband's anger and possible abandonment if she openly stated that she did not want another child to care for. Soon she realized that her weight kept her from having to confront her husband or deal with the issue at all. Her doctor had emphatically told her that having another child was far too dangerous an undertaking if she became pregnant at her current weight. Losing weight would mean confronting the issue and admitting the truth to her spouse. Once she realized this she knew that she would never let go of her extra pounds until she figured out how to handle this matter directly with her husband.

Scenarios like this one happen frequently as part of the therapy process. Women find out that their weight and out-of-control behavior provides them with illusions of safety. If women are overweight, they can avoid the situations that they fear. Women may think such thoughts as, "If I am heavy, men won't make advances towards me. If I am fat, I can't possibly_____(fill in the blank: go to school, ask for anything, be successful, take risks, compete with other women, have a good relationship, etc.). If I am obese, I'll be unattractive, other women won't be threatened by me and I'll have more friends. If I am fat, I won't be called upon to give my opinions or ideas. People won't take me seriously and I won't have to risk being wrong and feeling foolish. If I am overweight I may be excluded from good jobs where I will be expected to be responsible and competent (it is illegal, but it happens). If I am obese I can stay close to home—buses, planes, trains and subways have small seats so I can't possibly travel." This thinking provides an illusion of safety.

Being overweight is not simple and generally there are at least a few hidden, unconscious agendas behind the eating behavior. Close your eyes, take a few deep breaths and think for a few minutes about the advantages you get from being overweight. Then return to the present. Write those advantages down. Now note any other, more nurturing ways you can take care of yourself and your feelings and write these down. Next, choose one area where you would like to make a change. For example, if you have discovered that one advantage of overeating has been to numb feelings of grief, you might plan to talk with a friend about your loss. In this way, you allow your feelings to surface and find expression and you no longer need food to anesthetize yourself. You can do this exercise often as a way of checking in with yourself and changing your compulsive behavior.

ROBOTIC BEHAVIOR

Sometimes we eat and don't even realize we are eating—the biting, chewing and swallowing have become automatic. When we perform any behavior for a period of time, it becomes automatic. It is performed without conscious thought. Remember the first time you drove? You'd studied the traffic laws and watched the films in class. The first time you got behind the wheel and the instructor told you to start the car, you had to think of each detail. You had to pay close attention. You thought about putting the key into the ignition, placing your left foot on the clutch and your right one on the brake or gas, shifting into the appropriate gear, and then turning the key to the right. It felt strange and unfamiliar. It did not take long, however, for these behaviors to become automatic. Today, you most likely hop into your car and go without giving any of these details a conscious thought. You know how to drive. The motions have become automatic. Your subconscious is fully aware, however, to ensure you succeed at starting the car. And of course you must still be extremely conscious of being on the road and of other vehicles.

The same phenomenon takes place with our eating behavior and at a much younger age. As infants we cry for many reasons—perhaps we have an uncomfortable, wet diaper or a pain somewhere in our little body. We can't speak to tell our caretakers what is wrong and they often respond to our cries by putting a bottle or breast into our mouths. So we learn through this that crying brings us oral gratification. We quickly learn to associate food with comfort. We don't even have to think about it. It is automatic. We feel "bad," we reach for food. We experience discomfort of any kind, we eat.

As adults, if we feel "better" eating chocolate when we are upset about something, it doesn't take long for eating chocolate to become an automatic response when we want to feel better—and who doesn't frequently have times when they want to feel better? If we begin to eat snacks at night in front of our television sets, again, it can quickly become a thoughtless habit. Many women eat automatically when preparing meals for their families. They "taste" as they prepare supper and when the actual meal is ready, have already eaten more than enough. They then sit down with their family members and eat the full supper they have prepared for everybody else. The "before dinner food" was eaten automatically and barely noticed. They don't realize they have eaten the equivalent of two dinners and are truly surprised when the scale reflects their actions.

Another common situation in which people eat without consciousness is while driving. People who spend a lot of time on the road often find, if and when they notice, that they have been eating and eating and eating as they have been driving along. The snacking has become so *automatic* that it is virtually unnoticed. For most of us, food is readily accessible and easy to grab, especially fast foods and junk foods. Unhealthy food behaviors are easy to develop and impossible to change unless we are aware of them. How often do you "automatically" stop by the candy machine at work? How often do you eat and later feel surprised to notice you had eaten so much? How often do you engage in conversation with a dinner partner and finish your meal without having been aware of your food or the experience of eating? What are some of your patterns of automatic eating? Possibly you have been eating a great deal of food in this "robotic" way, barely noticing that you have been putting it into your mouth. Be assured, however, that although you may not be noticing what you are doing, your body *is* noticing, the calories are adding up, and your Chew is as happy as can be.

Sit down and think about times you may be engaging in robotic behavior. As you did in the previous section, close your eyes. Breathe deeply and think of ways you engage in robotic eating. Then return to the present and write down any automatic eating that you have become aware of. Next, make a plan to change one behavior. For example, if you realize that you have been munching while preparing dinner, make a choice to sip a large glass of lemon and water as you cook instead. In this way, you eliminate a behavior that is hazardous while substituting a healthy one. If you discover that you snack frequently while driving, choose not to bring food into your car anymore. Try this exercise often to see how many changes you can think of to make. Then make a plan to change them one at a time—*gradually* and *slowly*.

Another way to bring robotic eating into conscious awareness is to write down everything you eat during a one week period. Keeping a diary like this for a brief period can help you bring unconscious eating behavior into your conscious mind. A word of caution is necessary here. Do not keep a food diary longer than a few weeks. If you do, you may become more rigid and focused on food. You may find yourself more obsessed with your diet than ever. This is counterproductive, so use your diary briefly and *once you become aware of ways you have been using food automatically, you can make different choices.* Now that we have looked at some of the more common reasons for overeating, let's look in greater detail at some of the physical, emotional, social and spiritual causes of compulsive eating.

Reflections

CHAPTER II

Understanding the Physical Reasons for Overeating

MANY of us, perhaps particularly in the profession of psychology, fail to realize that overeating is only partly psychological, that there is a strong physical component to our behavior. Our clients may think, and we may join them in thinking, that if we can only find that one old emotional wound that needs healing or that one major conflict to solve, eating issues will magically disappear, as if that knowledge and that process *alone* are powerful enough to put a stop at last to the years of food-abusive behaviors.

It is true that much research has been done on the effects of various foods on our emotions. What does it mean *emotionally* if we eat too much or too little salt or fat? What happens inside our body if we choose only refined foods instead of whole foods? We may wonder why we race around in search of potato chips or chocolate with such fervor: what is our body trying to tell us that we are unable or unwilling to hear? Where can we acquire the knowledge we need to figure this out? In their best selling book, *Make the Connection,* Bob Greene and Oprah Winfrey offer clear explanations of some of the ways our body works. Some topics they address are: natural "set point" weight, water retention, ways we burn and store fat, metabolism, effects of different types of exercise and substances on our body and ways to manage compulsive eating behaviors and weight. Their presentation is clear and comprehensive and I highly recommend their book to learn more about these topics.

Not only do professionals lack knowledge of the physical reasons for overeating but society in general does as well. We are socialized to be preoccupied with weight and physical appearance and, in the process, we often cut ourselves off from our physical selves. We can maintain a negative image of our body within our subconscious mind while, in fact, having little actual awareness of ourselves as being in a body that feels and performs and moves about for us all day long. *Many women look in the mirror only from the neck up.* They apply creams and make up and often give little attention and nurturance to the rest of their beings. From the neck down is regarded as "the enemy"—that body which adamantly refuses to cooperate and conform to society's unrealistically thin image. How can we expect to love and care for our body if we detach from it and think of our body as an enemy?

Many of us also grew up in families where there was little awareness of healthy eating. The media encouraged our mothers to give us "love" by filling our lunchboxes with white bread and sugary cupcakes. One client told me that she had been raised by her grandmother who decorated cakes to make a living. Her grandmother had little money left over for healthy foods and my client would often be given the leftover cake tops and frosting (frosting sandwiches) for her dinner. In my home, we sometimes had what my mother named "assorted sandwiches." We loved this meal of little sandwich triangles (on white bread, of course) made from various jellies, butter, white sugar, marshmallow, molasses and peanut butter. Fortunately my mother did not feed us this very often. She did have nutritional common sense, but many mothers did not and many women suffer today with unhealthy habits left over from childhood.

Although many women come to see me having read nearly everything they could get their hands on regarding dieting, it is surprising that they often lack knowledge of the basics about food, nutrition and the effects of substances on their health and body size. These same women may also exercise with little understanding of the effects of movement on their bodies and they may view their bodies in distorted ways. I will take just a few moments here to consider some of these factors. This section is well worth spending time reading carefully. To change compulsive eating behavior, you must have basic knowledge about ways in which you are impacted by various foods and beverages, exercise and other physical factors. If you do not, you will continue to feel helpless and to eat in an out of control way

MOVING OUR BODIES

I grew up in a house with a large wooded area behind it. When I was small, I would run as fast as I could along the paths trying not to break a single twig or make a sound. I would run swiftly (like a deer, I thought). Sometimes I imagined I was an Indian princess or a brave running to save my village (I never knew from what). The wind would race past my ears. I would feel free and light as I hopped over tiny streams and logs. Moving was a game then. It was about having fun. Do you have a favorite memory of feeling comfortable like that in your body as a child? Many women do, but many do not, especially if they became physically self-conscious early on. For many of us though, moving stopped being fun at some time early in our lives.

I don't know when I stopped running like a deer, but at some point I did. Maybe I just got too busy with life and the business of paying attention to everyone else. Maybe I got self-conscious as I developed breasts. Maybe I realized that having fun being in my body was for "little kids" and I got too old for that sort of thing. I don't know. Whatever messages I did receive about my body did not encourage grace and speed unless they referred to competition or exhibition, like dancing class or team sports.

What I have noticed is that most women who come to see me have *abandoned their physical selves.* Our hearts beat, our breath enters and exits and we are oblivious. We generally do not take the time to acknowledge the miraculous tasks our bodies can perform. If we are not aware of what our bodies are doing, we will not cultivate appreciation for them and this lack of appreciation will make it even easier to abuse them. Conversely, if we take the time to notice and marvel at our wonderful bodies, we will be much more likely to attend to them with awe, compassion and love and it will be harder for us to abuse them.

Over the years we often become so focused on weight and appearance that we lose touch with the magic of our own movement. Also, our bodies mirror our emotions and if we feel rigid and tense, our bodies will likewise constrict. Moving our bodies is necessary if we are going to take care of ourselves. Remember, to achieve and maintain a reasonable weight, we must change our focus from how we look to how we feel. If we don't use our body, we can't appreciate it. If we don't appreciate it, we can't love and accept it. If we don't love and accept it, we will not take the steps necessary to nurture it. For many of us the thought of making friends with our body is frightening and sounds impossible. It is not.

We need to treat our body in a friendly way. Attending to ourselves in this fashion represents one part of a picture that is forming as we learn about our overeating behavior. To understand compulsive eating and to change old patterns, we must eventually look at the whole picture. Think of reading these preliminary sections as similar to looking at all the pieces of a jigsaw puzzle before you begin to fit them all together. In Part II, having spread out all the pieces and examined them, I will help you begin putting your own personal puzzle together. Then you will be putting a plan together for yourself to manage any compulsions to eat compulsively. *For now just know that moving your body is a central piece of this puzzle.*

THE CONFUSION OF BODY IMAGE

How do we see our physical selves? Most of us see our bodies unrealistically. Often we are not even aware of them. We can go through days and weeks never giving a conscious thought to our bodies. It is easy to take them for granted. We don't always pay attention to how our bodies feel and we don't view ourselves realistically. Try this: Stand in front of a mirror first thing in the morning before you have eaten anything and look at your body. Now, go eat a bite of something, like a cookie, and come back to the mirror. Do you look different? Does your body look noticeably *larger*? Most of us will see ourselves as larger than we did just moments before. Intellectually we may know that one small bite of food cannot double our weight in less than a minute, but our *perception* changes dramatically anyway. This is a clear example of distorted body image and most of us suffer with this to some degree.

Years ago I attended a cousin's wedding. She had cleverly taken old photographs of her guests and fashioned placecards for the tables from these photos. To find your seat, you needed to locate the old picture of yourself. This was fascinating to watch as guests roamed around searching for themselves. My experience was an eye-opener for me. I could not locate my own picture and my mother actually had to find it for me and direct me to my seat.

My cousin had used a picture of me that had been taken when I was in my late twenties—what I have come to call my "anorectic" days. I could not recognize the pale, thin image of myself at all! At first I protested that this was definitely not a likeness of me. The only way I became convinced that the picture I held really was of me was by recognizing the outfit I had been wearing at the time. I remembered my clothes and also recalled that I had felt quite fat at that time in my life! I would look in the mirror then with self-disgust and actually see an obese, pathetic person staring back at me. The memory of that image was in stark contrast to the emaciated image I held in my hand!

Many women report similar experiences. We cannot see ourselves objectively. Most of us look at pictures and see only the areas we are unhappy with (and in exaggerated ways). Our hips or bellies may look enormous to us at the time. Later, when we see the same pictures, we may see them differently. This depends upon how we are feeling about ourselves at that time. I often ask women who come to see me to bring in pictures of themselves as children and/or as adolescents. We look at these old photographs together and often women, who thought they were fat at the time, are able to see that they were, in fact, average weight children. For most this is a surprise and, for some, can open the door to looking in the mirror a bit less critically than they have in the past.

How we see ourselves has much to do with how we feel about ourselves. The more we focus on the negative in our lives, the more negatively we will view images of ourselves. Later in this book, we will address the importance of changing negative attitudes to positive ones. *For now, just know that our perceptions of ourselves can be grossly inaccurate and that they change as our feelings about ourselves change.*

APPRECIATING LIFE CHANGES

We are always evolving from one stage of life to another, from one body shape to another. We travel over time from babies to little girls, to adolescents, to women, to elders. These life passages happen gradually and have profound effects on the ways we view and care for our physical bodies. Do you recall when you first noticed your developing breasts or when your pubic hair began to appear? Do you remember when you first began to menstruate? Some of you remember going through the bodily changes that accompany pregnancy and birth. Others know what it was like to negotiate the often stormy waters of menopause. How did you react to these changes? How did your feelings towards your body change over time? Were you fearful, excited, curious, anxious, or ashamed? Did you talk to anyone about the changes you were noticing or did you struggle with unanswered questions all by yourself?

Many women report that they felt confused and lonely through these life changes and most women agree that certain life changes were a least somewhat disturbing to them. As we mature our bellies are *supposed* to become round and our hips full but society tells us they are not. So, as our bodies change in natural ways throughout our lives, we may see ourselves in negative ways—as fat, unacceptable, unattractive. It is nearly impossible to feel good about ourselves and our bodies in this culture. Most women's bodies could never match those we are taught to view as ideal and even women who have achieved this look are often frightened that they will be unable to maintain their thin appearance over time. For a number of my clients, maintaining weight loss has proven far more difficult and stressful than achieving the weight loss in the first place.

It is no wonder that so many of us have been struggling with compulsive eating behaviors for years. Here are these bodies we received at birth behaving in ways that we have no control over. We cannot stop our chests from developing any more than we can stop our hair from growing or the sun from coming up. Yet we punish our bodies for simply doing what they are supposed to do. We want to look different than we look—be taller, thinner, have curly hair or a different tone to our skin. *Part of stopping compulsive eating behavior permanently means accepting each bodily change as a natural part of life and ourselves as exactly who we're supposed to be.* We will talk more about the issue of societal expectations and the difficulty of accepting ourselves fully in Part I, Chapter IV.

APPEARANCE OR COMFORT

Have you ever stopped to pay attention to the ways men and women are expected to dress? I'm not talking about casual wear.

Fortunately, much of that is "gender friendly." I am talking about clothes for work, for a date, for the office or an evening out, for example. Have you ever looked at a fashion magazine and compared images of both genders? The men are seen standing comfortably in some combination of pants and shirts or jackets. Women, on the other hand, are often found in various uncomfortable positions balancing precariously on shoes with high heels that offer no support to their feet.

These women frequently appear in tight skirts or dresses and, unless they are as thin as pencils, they may have tight undergarments on that pinch when they exhale. In some outfits women look and feel constricted. The clothes they have on just don't fit. Now this is a sensitive area for some people and I am not saying there is anything wrong with wearing the latest styles. What I *am* saying is that some of these styles are not a comfortable choice of clothing for many of us. It is hard for us to relax and feel okay about being ourselves. In clothes that make us uncomfortable on the outside it is even harder for us to feel comfortable on the inside.

For years, many of us have tried, usually with little or no success, to portray a certain image and we have been brainwashed into looking outside of ourselves to decide exactly what that image is. We have been told how to dress and how to feel about it. I recall being in seventh grade and feeling simultaneously excited and nervous about starting ballroom dancing classes. Shortly before the first lesson, my mother presented me with a garter belt, nylon stockings, a girdle and a long line bra. Imagine that! Seventh grade and already I had to fuss to hide every bulge and jiggle. My emotions, as I recall, were mixed. Partly I was excited to make my grand entrance into this mysterious grown up world and partly I was horrified. I remember the flesh of my thighs overflowing the tight little stocking tops and I remember smiling through my misery as I tried to look absolutely beautiful gliding across the dance floor. What was to be a magical, wonderful experience turned into a strained and difficult one. Did you ever find yourself in such a predicament? Were you ever dressed to match an image that didn't quite fit?

We do not live in a culture where we are encouraged to be creative. We do not celebrate differences in body shapes, sizes and styles and we do not learn to love and appreciate our bodies as unique and beautiful no matter how large or small. Instead, for the majority of us, we are shown how to hide our curves and "flaws." This is unfortunate. Our self-esteem certainly suffers and we might go through our entire lives feeling unacceptable, inadequate, unattractive, constricted and ashamed.

A number of years ago I attended a women's music festival in Michigan. Thousands of women attended the week-long event and no men were permitted on the festival land. The summer weather was deliciously warm most of the time and the majority of the women wore little, if any, clothing during the day. All ages were represented. There were little girls and elders, and there were women from many different countries. I saw women of all shapes, sizes and colors. These women walked freely about the land and appearance mattered little. I thought what a beautiful sight it was to see these women moving about freely, uninhibited by social expectations or clothing constraints.

Now I know we can't all walk around without our clothes on. Nor would we want to. Buying and wearing clothes that please us is fun. We can choose colors and materials that we love and think of our own needs when we purchase clothing. We can dress for comfort and still look stylish. One of the reasons we may overeat is because we fall short in our vain attempts to look like the models we see. If we try to emulate these women, who are perpetually young and unrealistically thin, nearly all of us will fail. *Please do not dress to look like or be someone else. Be yourself. Be comfortable and breathe. Choose what suits you.*

SOME HARMFUL SUBSTANCES

The media is full of recommendations presented by people who profess to be sincerely interested in giving us good advice based on "the latest research" and our primary source of information often is television, magazines, the internet and radio. The problem is that different people tell us different things based on the way they have interpreted the data (often skewing things to support their own self-interests or the interests of those financing their research). Information for this section was taken from books by contemporary writers in the Alternative Health field. These references can be found in the reading list at the back of this book. You will find titles by Andrew Weil, M.D., Harvey and Marilyn Diamond, Christiane Northrup, M.D., Amadea Morningstar, and Annemarie Colbin particularly useful if you wish to read more about how your body is affected by the substances I will mention. I encourage you to read these and to do additional research on your own. The more fully informed you are, the more you empower yourself with that knowledge, the more you will be able to take control of your health and your weight. Following is a short list of substances and some of the ways they harm our moods and our bodies. This section is brief. I include it to give you a sense of the effects some foods and beverages have on your body and on your intention to stop compulsive eating behavior.

Alcohol

In his book *Natural Health, Natural Medicine* Andrew Weil, M.D. addresses alcohol use: "Heavy alcohol use puts us at risk of developing cancers of the mouth, throat, esophagus, and stomach, probably because alcohol irritates these tissues directly." Weil also states that heavy drinkers are more likely to get liver cancer and that this danger is compounded if you also smoke tobacco. He recommends drinking moderately or minimally or not at all.

Besides the physiological dangers of alcohol use, there are psychological dangers as well. Many women report that after drinking, they feel out of control, are more likely to throw out their plans to eat sensibly and to binge. Alcohol weakens their resolve to restrict "forbidden" foods and drinking often precipitates weeks or months of "out of control" behavior. This behavior is accompanied by feelings of remorse, guilt and self-disgust which can lead the drinker to drink or eat even more in an attempt to "medicate" these negative feelings.

The Diamonds report that alcohol impairs calcium absorption by affecting the liver's ability to activate vitamin D which is important in the metabolism of calcium. Christiane Northrup, M.D. associates excess alcohol consumption with increased risk of breast cancer, menstrual irregularities, osteoporosis and birth defects. She also explains that "two drinks of alcohol per night effectively wipe out rapid eye movement (REM) sleep, which is the type of sleep associated with dreaming." She wisely points out that dreaming is part of our internal guidance system and wonders why anyone would choose to suppress that guidance with alcohol. Consensus of opinion appears to be that alcohol offers no beneficial effects. You decide.

Artificial Sweeteners

At the Psychology of Health, Immunity and Disease Conference at Hilton Head, South Carolina, Annemarie Colbin, author of *Food and Healing*, warned her audience of the dangers of ingesting the artificial sweetener, aspartame. Colbin stated that this sweetener, found in so many popular diet products, has been linked to hypoglycemia, disturbed thyroid function, excess phenylalanine, and possible blockage of serotonin (the calming chemical). It has been associated with increased craving for sweets, irritability, tingling of the extremities, mild to suicidal depression, insomnia, hostility, anxiety, inability to cope, memory loss, seizures, personality and mood changes. She recommends using only whole, natural sweeteners such as maple syrup or barley malt in your diet.

Andrew Weil, M.D. in his book *Natural Health, Natural Medicine* reports that he has seen many women who have suffered headaches and aggravated premenstrual symptoms as a result of aspartame use. He also comments on other artificial sweeteners in his book and states we are better off using moderate amounts of sugar than putting ourselves at risk with any artificial sweetening products. Deepak Chopra, M.D., author of *Perfect Weight* states that honey is not only acceptable but is a beneficial addition to the diet. He claims that a small amount of honey taken periodically throughout the day can decrease sugar cravings and increase metabolism. The consensus is that if you must use a sweetener, natural is best. Choose maple syrup, barley malt, honey or stevia.

Isn't it truly amazing how willing many of us have been to take in "diet" foods with little or no concern for the adverse ways which they may affect our health? Most women I have worked with have entirely overlooked the dangerous effects of no-fat or sugar-free foods. They see these instead as *magic* foods that they can eat to excess. Usually, they end up eating an overabundance of these "poison" foods and less whole, nutritious ones. The more we turn to "dead," processed foods and avoid "live" whole foods, the more our moods and appetites become affected and the more we are likely to compensate with a binge.

Caffeine

Coffee, chocolate, non-herbal tea, some medications and many soft drinks contain caffeine. Caffeine initially speeds up body systems and many women claim they enjoy this "rush" because they experience temporary energy and can more easily go without solid food— having a cup of coffee instead of a nutritional breakfast. Mistakenly, they think they are helping themselves by taking in fewer calories and consequently losing weight. This is an illusion. Caffeine can produce anxiety. For some of us anxiety can be the catalyst to compulsive eating, especially of non-nutritional foods. For others, it can precipitate powerful urges to withhold nourishment. If you react to anxiety by withholding food, you give your body the message that it is in danger and your body decides it must store the calories and fats it has to prevent starvation. This is an example of our primal fear of famine kicking in. Even though our intellect knows there is no chance of actual starvation, our body has its own set of instructions left over from millions of years ago when food was difficult to obtain.

Caffeine intake leads to irritability and anxiety. Because our metabolism is accelerated, our body is working much harder than it needs to and we become exhausted. Caffeine can precipitate panic attacks and heart palpitations. It also acts as a diuretic and causes our bodies to excrete twice as much calcium as we normally would. Excessive use of it can lead to dehydration. Since thirst is often mistaken for hunger, the dehydration effect can also lead to overeating. So, physically, caffeine use is self-abusive and may mislead us into thinking we are gaining energy and getting smaller by eliminating fluids. What is really happening, however, is that we are exhausting our body, lowering our metabolism by withholding food, increasing our anxiety and assuring that weight control and optimum health are *harder* to achieve.

As previously mentioned, anxiety caused by excessive caffeine intake can lead many of us straight to the doughnut shop or candy store to get what we think we need to calm our nerves (mask our feelings). So using caffeine leads many of us to seek out fats and sugars which provide temporary satisfaction and relief while, at the same time, assuring us of a lowered metabolism, increased anxiety, decreased energy and increased fat storage. Many of us also end up feeling exhausted and depressed as the effects of caffeine wear off and we may crave more caffeine. What a *not*-so-merry-go-round!

A favorite caffeine choice for many women is chocolate (particularly just prior to menstruation). This substance contains caffeine and also theobromine (which acts in a similar way to caffeine) and is a powerful, mood altering, addictive drug. People joke about being "chocoholics" but, for many, this topic is not a laughing matter. What eating chocolate does is provide sugar, fat and caffeine. It is a perfect binge food!

Dairy

At the Psychology of Health, Immunity and Disease Conference at Hilton Head, South Carolina Annemarie Colbin shared an interesting theory regarding the use of dairy products by adults in our culture. According to Ms. Colbin, drinking milk and eating dairy are signs that the adult in question has never really been weaned. She hypothesized that turning to milk may give us some of the oral gratification and nurturing feelings we crave. Harvey and Marilyn Diamond share a similar view in their book, *Fit for Life II*. They state that milk is not essential to the human diet and they point out that no other species of animal (in the wild) consumes milk of another species and, once weaned, no animal ever again consumes milk. They posit that "cows don't drink cows milk, so why do humans?" Andrew Weil, M.D. in his work, *Natural Health, Natural Medicine* wrote, "Milk probably is nature's most perfect food for baby cows, but not for human beings." Christiane Northrup, M.D. in her book *Women's Bodies, Women's Wisdom* points out that three-quarters of the world's population maintains health without drinking milk after infancy. Then why do so many people consider milk a healthy, nourishing choice?

We have been given powerful messages all of our lives through the media, our schools and our families about drinking our milk and we may be experiencing false security about using dairy products. We may think we are being good to our bodies, taking in essential vitamins and minerals and protecting ourselves from osteoporosis. Some of you may even remember watching television and toasting President Eisenhower with a big glass of milk along with Big Brother Bob Emery in the 1950's. I know I did and drinking milk felt not only healthy but also patriotic at the time. It was the *right* thing to do. Following is a brief synopsis of what some contemporaries in the Holistic Health field are saying about dairy; however, keep in mind that new studies are being conducted all the time. Information we receive today may be vastly different from what is reported tomorrow.

Andrew Weil, M.D., Harvey and Marilyn Diamond and

Christiane Northrup, M.D. all report that milk is implicated in the development of numerous physical complaints. I refer you to works by these authors in the reading section of this book for detailed information. Weil, The Diamonds and Northrup also all address the myth that we need milk as a calcium source. According to them, our calcium should come from grains, green leafy vegetables, kale, collard greens, broccoli, raw nuts, raw sesame seeds (particularly high in calcium), most fruits, kelp, dulse, molasses, tofu, and concentrated fruits such as figs, dates and prunes. This is a controversial topic, however, and the National Osteoporosis Foundation does recommend that besides other calcium rich foods, women include skim milk and cheese in their diet. It is up to you to educate yourself, weigh all the information you gather, listen to your inner voice of wisdom and make the choices that make most sense to you.

Amadea Morningstar, author of a wonderful book entitled *Ayurvedic Cooking for Westerners,* and Paavo Airola who wrote *Are You Confused?* mention that milk has played a significant role in the diet of many health conscious people in centuries past and was considered of therapeutic value before the days of pasteurization. Both, however, state that the milk presently obtainable by the consumer is not helpful to health. Both agree that for milk to be a viable nutrition source, it must come from healthy animals raised on organic farms where no chemical fertilizers are used. It must be raw, unpasturized, free from chemical additives and any residues of drugs, hormones, antibiotics, detergents and pesticides, and should be consumed within 24 hours of the milking. Obtaining milk of this quality in such a timely fashion is impossible for most of us. This makes drinking milk out of the question for the majority of us. If you are used to using milk regularly try substituting soy or rice milk instead.

Salt

Salt is found in animal products and added to much of our food by the companies who process it. In addition, many people pour salt directly onto their foods. Andrew Weil, M.D. considers the effects of salt thoroughly in his book, *Natural Health, Natural Medicine.* According to him, salt may be harmful for some people and not so for others. He states that most of us consume much more salt than our bodies require. According to Weil, excessive consumption of salt can lead to abnormally high blood pressure, (hypertension) and resultant strokes, congestive heart failure, kidney disease, fluid retention (edema, bloating), and headaches. Harvey and Marilyn Diamond add: "The more sodium (salt) you take in, the more calcium you excrete." Colbin points out that, in addition to these consequences, high salt intake leads to increased stress. (Any increase in our stress level can prompt us to quickly forge a trail straight to the refrigerator!) Given this, it appears that using salt sparingly and prudently is fine for most of us. Stay away, however, from foods to which much salt has been added and do not add salt to your food. A little salt goes a long way!

Sugar

Sugar is an interesting substance. It is extremely addictive for many people and many women report that if they have one bite of a sugary food it precipitates a binge. There are a number of psychological reasons for feeling out of control after eating sugar and I will discuss some of these in the section of this book dealing with emotional components of compulsive eating, but for now let's consider what happens on a purely physical level. When we take sugar into our systems, a series of events occurs. Our blood sugar level rises quickly and our body begins to manufacture insulin. Adrenaline floods our system and our heart rate increases. Our blood pressure goes up and we feel "high." This "high" feeling doesn't last long, however, and soon our blood sugar level drops causing our body to beg and plead for more sugar and more "energy."

When this happens we may feel exhausted, irritable and depressed. If you experience mood swings, mental dullness or become tired easily, try eliminating sugar from your diet for a week. You will most likely notice a significant reduction of all of these symptoms. This is the physical process everyone experiences when eating sugar—not only when bingeing. It is as simple as that but many women do not realize that eating sugar can cause such powerful, often irresistible physical cravings. Additionally, eating sugar dulls emotion and women function as if they have no feelings.

The reality is there is no "final verdict" on the use of any of the foods or beverages mentioned here. This makes it difficult to sort out facts from myths. We can only do what we can to educate ourselves and make the best choices we can based on the knowledge we have.

As we approach the end of this section it is important to note Annemarie Colbin's position that we are each unique and have different, individual needs. For each of us eating too little of certain foods can be just as problematic as eating too much. In her lecture at the Psychology of Health, Immunity and Disease Conference, Colbin stated that anger is often linked to either too much or too little fat and that we need a bit of olive oil or organic butter in our diets. She also pointed out that too much water may increase anxiety and that either too much or too little salt can cause fear (common in people with phobias). Excess sweets are associated with worry, depression, melancholy and fear. Not eating enough protein can make us tired. Too few carbohydrates can make people "uptight." Excess or lack of spicy, stimulating foods can be connected to anxiety, grief and sadness. For each of us the amounts of various foods we need differ and we must each experiment to find the optimal amounts of foods we feel best eating. In her book *Food and Healing,* Colbin includes a useful chart showing how different foods affect us emotionally and suggests foods we may choose to counteract the undesirable effects of our diet. She also shares her knowledge of various diets and much useful information about cooking and balancing food. I highly recommend this book if you would like to expand your knowledge in this area.

Paying attention to what we put into our bodies and how it affects us physically, emotionally and spiritually is of great importance. I frequently suggest to clients that they eliminate sugar and caffeine from their diet for a brief period of time before we begin therapy. I explain symptoms they might experience as they eliminate these "poisons" from their systems (e.g. headaches, weakness, diarrhea) and I offer them support through this detoxification period. I encourage them to be particularly gentle with themselves at this time and to attend to their spiritual selves as well (e.g. through meditation, journal writing or spending time in nature). Sometimes these people find that these dietary changes are all that is necessary to help them feel better. Therapy is not automatically the best course of treatment.

There are not always psychological reasons for compulsive eating behaviors. At times there are, but not in all cases. Once a woman has rid her body of most harmful substances, she is able to sort out physical complaints from those of a psychological or spiritual nature. (Perhaps if we all ate more consciously there would be little demand for anti-depressants or anti-anxiety medications.) If, after cleansing, my client and I agree that some form of psychotherapy would be helpful, we continue meeting. Because the physical reasons for her overeating have already been addressed, she is able to think more clearly and this frees us to explore other areas of her life in which she is experiencing distress.

Consider cutting down on or eliminating sugar and caffeine from your diet for a period of time and see how you feel after a few weeks. You may be very pleasantly surprised. Be prepared, however, that you may feel tired for the first week or so and may experience other detoxification symptoms, such as headaches. If you want to stop taking caffeine, cut down gradually to minimize withdrawal symptoms. If you eliminate sugar you are likely to crave it for a few days. Drink lots of water to flush your system, get plenty of rest and exercise moderately. The cravings should disappear in two to three days. Notice how you feel emotionally and physically when you eat or drink different substances. Learn as much as you can about yourself and your relationship with foods and beverages in this way. *Be aware. Educate yourself. Make the changes that make the most sense to you.*

Reflections

CHAPTER III

*U*nderstanding the *E*motional *R*easons for *O*vereating

PSYCHOLOGICALLY, food issues are complex. Women come to see me because I am a psychologist and a Doctor of Holistic Health and they are interested in understanding why they choose to eat to excess. Most have been battling with compulsive eating issues for years and are truly *exhausted* and *desperate*. They come wanting to understand themselves in order to change self-destructive behaviors once and for all. For a few, making dietary changes alone will help them feel better. For most, the situation is more complicated. *Women know instinctively, if not consciously, that successful weight loss and maintenance depends upon understanding and resolving the feelings they "avoid" by numbing themselves with food.* We always talk about this in one of our first meetings.

For most of us the battle began early on. We may or may not recall when we first began to abuse food, but we know that self-destructive, uncontrolled eating has become a central, and often shameful, part of our lives. We may have had relatives who commented upon our body size or mothers who monitored what we put into our mouths. I know, personally, that my own mother must have possessed magical powers. She was able to hear me chewing anything from several rooms away. If I took a cookie from the kitchen and retreated to my room to eat it, her voice would echo down the hall. "Do you need it, Denise?" My mother meant well. She loved me and she was trying to help me to be slender and attractive but I could not appreciate her effort. Instead I would flood with embarrassment and shame and yearn for even more cookies to medicate my anxiety. Oh the power of these old experiences! Can you recall any?

In this chapter we will look at some of the emotional components of our out of control behavior. You are likely to recognize parts of yourself on these pages and some unpleasant memories may be evoked. Please read on with an open and gentle heart. This section may provoke anxiety, anger, sadness or other feelings. Try to welcome these feelings and remind yourself that experiencing all of your feelings is a natural and beneficial part of healing and moving on. You are not alone. We are all together in our struggle to understand.

THE MOTHER/DAUGHTER CONNECTION

The mother/daughter bond is a complex one. It is important to think about it and to understand it if we are to make sense of our compulsive eating behavior. Many women report that they learned dieting behaviors from their mothers, who were themselves often obsessed with food and weight. If one female child in the family was affected, often any other females were as well. It is not uncommon to find one sister obese, one anorectic and one bulimic, for example. Some of my clients report mothers taking them to places like Diet Workshop or Weight Watchers while the mother attended meetings. This often established a bond between the two and, for many women, that became a central part of their relationship with their mother. Mothers and daughters went on diets together, overate together and worried together as they gained weight. They shared the shame and the guilt and, in many cases, grew larger and larger together.

I recall, as a child of twelve or so, taking a diet drink called Metrecal with my mother and sister. This was a milkshake-type concoction in chocolate or vanilla. We would all sit down together four times a day and have one of these shakes as our meal. This was not too bad for the first few "meals" but soon the lack of solid food began to feel like torture. My memory is that the time spent together was wonderful, but the focus was negative. We reminded ourselves four times a day that our bodies were not as they should be and that we needed to starve ourselves into a shape we were not meant to have. Needless to say, we lasted only a short time and eventually we each gained back more than we had lost when the deprivation ended.

Can you recall similar experiences? Did you eat truckloads of grapefruits or drink gallons of water in vain attempts to attain the slender body which is held as the only standard of beauty in our culture? Was your mother dieting too? Did you diet with her to please her or to take care of her? Did you join with her in hopes of winning her approval and having something in common to share? Did you talk about body size, calories, weight and diets? Has that old behavior now become a central part of your own life? Was any of this behavior part of the bond you and your mother shared? If so, it is time to discard old assumptions and break these old patterns. We will explore ways to do this as we move through the second half of this book.

A LOOK AT SELF-ESTEEM

Low self-esteem is always present when we are trapped in a cycle of food abusive behavior. Why is it so hard to feel good about ourselves? Why do so many of us have such poor self-esteem? To answer this, we must examine what self-esteem is, how negative self-esteem develops and what we need to do to improve it. Self-esteem is not solid. It is fluid. Many people think of it as something that "just is." You may have heard someone remark that they have high or low self-esteem and that is the end of it. Well, it really isn't that way. Think of self-esteem as a river. Sometimes there is plenty of water in it and it flows freely. We may see sun sparkles reflected in it and it is quite beautiful. At other times, the water in our river may be quite low and we see mud, old tires and rusty things sticking up—not very attractive!

Self-esteem is like this river. It is high at times, low at others. Water flows into the river through positive messages we receive from ourselves and from others. Water flows out, however, when we hear and absorb negative messages. Think about this. When we were children, our parents expended a great deal of energy to take care of us. Since they had a limited amount of energy and wanted us to grow up doing the "right" things, they usually focused more attention on us when we were doing something wrong. If we were doing something unacceptable, that behavior had to be corrected. If we were not, there was no need to say anything to us.

Unfortunately, for many of us, the negative messages composed the bulk of what we heard. If we failed to do the dishes or take out the garbage, most likely we heard about it. Seldom though did one of our parents complement us for making our bed or doing our chores. If we were doing what was expected, it was usually taken for granted. Our parents may not have thought to compliment us or they may not have had the energy. Only when we didn't behave perfectly was our behavior commented on because our parents had an interest in having us change it.

For some of us, our parents may have focused on the negative to the exclusion of the positive. Did you ever, for example, bring home a report card with several high grades and one low one? Did your parents react to the positive ones or did they ask why the low grade? If they questioned the low grade, chances are they were raised the same way that they raised you. You may have learned, by receiving this negative attention, to treat yourself in the same harsh way. When you make a mistake, for example, do you "beat yourself up" for doing so? How often do you stop to praise yourself when you have done something well? It is a mighty task to feel good about ourselves following a childhood fraught with negative messages.

Damaging messages not only came from our caretakers but also from many other sources as well. As we will examine closely in the section dealing with socialization, we are surrounded by messages about our shortcomings. These can harm us again and again if we allow them to. In Part II, we will look at ways to improve self-esteem and to feel better about ourselves. If we try to lose weight without learning to appreciate ourselves, we will fail again and again. *Self-acceptance and self-love are absolutely essential.*

THE IMPACT OF ABUSE

Child abuse plays a significant role for numerous women who struggle with eating difficulties. Many of us suffered some form of abuse during our childhood or adolescence. We may have been beaten, ridiculed, ignored, sexually violated, or made to feel inferior or damaged in some way. For some of us, the abusive behavior was blatant. For others, it was subtle. In fact, women I am working with often report that unless the abuse they experienced was obvious and severe they have no right to feel angry or badly about ways they were treated. If their bones weren't broken or they weren't bleeding and bruised, they minimize the incidents of abusive behavior. Commonly, a pattern of circular thinking ensues. They may think: What is wrong with *me* that *I* was such a "bad" child? What did *I* do to deserve to be treated so poorly? How did *I* cause my abuse?

As children we depend on the adults in our world to meet our basic needs. We rely on them for food, clothing, shelter, protection, security and love. Each of us is born with a right to have these needs met. This means emotionally, physically, socially, spiritually and intellectually. When a parent fails to meet our needs, to protect us or to treat us with love and respect, we cannot optimally thrive. As babies we are tiny and powerless. We depend on trusted adults for nurturance and cannot make sense out of the world on our own.

No parents are perfect. We all make mistakes (just as our parents did) and cannot attend to everything for every child—we are torn between raising children and providing for them; between caring for children and molding them. The responsibilities of parenthood are enormous and we may enter adulthood ill-equipped to handle them (as our parents may also have been). We may be uncertain about how to best nurture our children. We may not know how to express our love freely while maintaining the boundaries necessary for good parenting. Children require their caretakers to demonstrate their love for them in order to learn that they are lovable. They need to experience this love through the eyes, voice and manner of those who attend to them. If a child fails to receive these messages of love and approval from their caretakers, they will not feel lovable and acceptable and their self-esteem will be diminished.

We may have received many negative messages about ourselves both verbally and non-verbally, both subtly and openly. Our self-esteem may have been trampled again and again. It is hard to feel good about ourselves when we are small and dependent upon others to teach us how to operate successfully in the world. Childhood and adolescence are times of turmoil and confusion. They need to be. We are rapidly growing, changing and trying to figure out how to fit into the world on our own—how to be. When we turn to our parents for help with this process and ask for their guidance, encouragement and support and do not consistently receive what we need, we suffer consequences. Our self-esteem is negatively affected.

It is common for women who come to see me with food control issues to recall histories of parents or others who physically, emotionally or sexually abused them. Many came from blatantly dysfunctional families where they felt isolated and emotionally abandoned. Self-destructive eating behaviors may have developed then as one available way to cope with the feelings of guilt, alienation and shame that are a result of being victimized in any way. If parents or others were abusive towards us, we may consider ourselves responsible (it is sometimes too frightening to realize that your caretakers are not doing their job). Remember, many of us learned to use food to soothe ourselves in times of stress. This behavior is persistent and it is hard (but by no means impossible) to learn new ways to cope with these painful feelings. You can learn to soothe yourself without eating compulsively!

It is essential to know, and to believe deep down in your adult heart of hearts, that you were not responsible for any abuse you suffered as a child. Children simply are not responsible. Adults are. If anyone treated you with disrespect, if any adult hurt you in any way, shame on them. You were just trying to survive. You were trying to make sense of the world and to negotiate your way through it. You are not "bad" now and you were not "bad" then. No matter what the circumstances were, any abuse of any kind that occurred was the fault of the adult or adults involved. If the abuse was by an older child, the fault still does not lie with you. An older child who performs abusive behavior has most likely been the recipient of abuse him or herself. The fault lies with those who influenced his or her life.

If you are *currently* being abused physically or emotionally, I urge you to read one or two of the many books currently available about domestic violence. *You do not need to stay in any situation that is harmful to you.* There are people with whom you can speak confidentially who will help you to get out of any abusive situation. I suggest you call The National Domestic Abuse Hotline (see the Resources section of this book) and read Marian Betancourt's book *What to Do when Love Turns Violent.*

Unfortunately, many of us who felt out of control as children carry with us the fear and anxiety that we experienced then. Even though we are in adult bodies now and we do have the ability to meet our own needs, we may still feel powerless and inadequate, most notably in times of stress. If we were victimized as children or are being victimized today, we may perceive ourselves as victims. If we felt "out of control" as children, we may easily feel "out of control" today. Feelings that linger from childhood experiences may interfere with our ability to take control of our lives as adults. They may sabotage even our best efforts to feel in control of our eating behavior in the present.

If you have been carrying the burden of shame and guilt, please consider seeking the services of a caring therapist who is experienced with abuse issues and who can help you to break the self-destructive patterns you may have developed as a result of your victimization. It is critically important to attend to this issue to truly free yourself from compulsive, self-destructive behaviors. It takes courage and commitment to talk about old, painful experiences in order to move through the shame and guilt associated with abuse but it is time and effort well spent. By releasing the past, you empower yourself in the present and you free yourself from the anxiety of feeling like a victim. Letting go of anxiety and empowering yourself are major actions which will help you eliminate the need to soothe yourself with food and to step away naturally from the need to eat compulsively. Your Chew will tell you that you must always be a victim and that you can never be free. Your Chew is *wrong*. You can be and you deserve to be free. You are worthy of this.

FOOD AND FEELINGS

For many of us food has been a trusted friend, a comfort. When we feel lonely or afraid or sad, food is always there. We use it to mask our difficult feelings and to nurture ourselves. We can count on it. In the moment, it does not let us down. When we use food as a comfort, however, the result is usually discomfort. We feel disappointed in ourselves and beat ourselves up emotionally with negative messages. When we have binged and feel exhausted, we vow never to abuse food again. Of course, the next time difficult feelings arise, we do. We do this because we have learned that "food works" and we have reinforced that again and again over the years. So, food works in the short term but in the long term overeating reinforces our negative self-image, lowers our self-esteem level and confirms again that we are out of control. We cannot change this behavior until we learn healthy ways to cope with difficult feelings.

Where did any of us ever get the idea that we should feel good all the time? When a feeling comes along that we experience as unpleasant, we think something must be wrong and we have to get rid of that uncomfortable feeling right away. We try to figure out what's wrong—which usually means *what we have done wrong*—so we can correct it and feel good again. Not only is it dreadfully hard work to try to "feel good" all the time, it is impossible. All human beings, at times, have feelings of dread, sadness, worthlessness, shame, envy, etc.

It is time to do something constructive with our feelings and to stop futilely trying to eliminate them. We can learn to sit with our feelings and to pay attention to the messages our feelings are trying to communicate. Both our pleasant and unpleasant feelings are valuable to us. They tell us much about ourselves. To eliminate them without first attending to the messages they bring is not useful and keeps us on a treadmill, eating to soothe ourselves with no idea why. You will find helpful exercises in Part II, and resources in the reading list at the back of this book. These will help you learn constructive ways to recognize feelings and to pay attention to the information they bring. Only then will you be able to handle these feelings in appropriate ways—not by stuffing and numbing yourself with food.

We need to think of our feelings as messages to us about ourselves and about our world and to accept each of these feelings as useful. This does not mean accepting abusive, unhealthy situations or relationships in our lives. If we feel uncomfortable because of someone or something we clearly need to confront, then the uncomfortable feeling has served as a message to deal with a situation. Until we do, the situation remains the same and our uncomfortable feelings, and urges to eat, persist. *Learning to attend to and accept our feelings is an essential factor in cultivating healthy eating behaviors.*

Not only do we turn to food when unpleasant feelings occur. We may also seek comfort and gratification from food, based on pleasant life experiences. Let me share an example with you from my own life. When I was a tiny child, perhaps only three or four, I would sometimes spend time with my grandmother. She would be busy cleaning and cooking and so forth and I would be nearby at play. In her neighborhood there was a baker who traveled from house to house in a small van. Occasionally, he would stop at my grandmother's when I was visiting and she would look over his tray of goods. After looking over all of his wares, she would inevitably choose a box of huge, plain doughnuts (my favorite). When the baker left, my grandmother would call me to her. She would put two doughnuts on the table and two glasses of orange juice and we would sit together and talk. This was an important time for me. My grandmother would focus all of her loving attention on me and, for a brief time, I would feel important, special, connected and loved. Is it any wonder that today when I feel disconnected, lonely or "not-so-special," that I experience a powerful urge to fill myself up with doughnuts and orange juice? Can you recall certain foods that were special to you during your early years? Were there certain people you felt close to or happy with that you shared eating experiences with? What did you share? Notice what you are feeling next time you crave that particular food.

One client who had an insatiable appetite for vanilla ice cream told me the following story. When she was a little girl her family would go out on hot, summer weekends to a local dairy bar for ice cream. Her mother would always ask her what flavor she preferred and she would always reply, "vanilla." Her mother would urge her to get something else, like butter pecan or maple walnut, claiming that she could have vanilla anytime at home. My client remained firm, however, and insisted upon vanilla. As a small child, there were not many opportunities for her to be assertive, make decisions and to have control over anything. She became aware through telling this story that her cravings for vanilla ice cream were closely connected to her need for control in her life. When she craved the ice cream she could ask herself what she needed to do to take care of herself and to regain control. Usually she could identify areas of her life where she was not asserting herself. By attending to these areas, she often was able to pass by the dairy bar and not act on the craving.

We use food to deal with feelings. For example, we may choose creamy foods to soothe hurt feelings and crunchy ones to suppress anger. Notice what foods you crave. Keep a journal with you and note what foods you eat. This information can help you to get more in touch with feelings you may be trying to deny or suppress. Most of us learned to hide our feelings and to attend more to others' feelings. As a result, it may be scary to speak out at first. We fear we will hurt someone else's feelings, provoke their anger, or cause them to leave us. Fears such as these keep us silent and food helps us maintain the silence. You will learn more about communicating and asserting yourself in *Healing the Emotional Self* in Part II.

THE IMPORTANCE OF CONNECTION

Connection is a basic human need. It is through our relationships with others that we learn about ourselves. As infants, we need connection and touch to teach us that we are lovable. We need connections to thrive and to grow. (You may be familiar with studies in which baby monkeys failed to thrive when they received no touch or contact.) This need does not evaporate as we mature. Deep within each of us exists a core of love and we yearn to express this with others. We will explore this core of love further in Part II, Chapter V, *Healing the Spiritual Self.* For now it is only important to realize that to attend to ourselves, we also must attend to others and we need others to attend to us. *We must feel a flow, a give and take, of loving energy in our lives in order to thrive and to feel good about ourselves.* This is particularly true of women.

Much research about women and relationships has been conducted by Jean Baker Miller, M.D., and her colleagues at the Stone Center at Wellesley College in Wellesley, Massachusetts. Dr. Miller and several other women began meeting early in the 1970's to think and talk about how women relate to themselves, others and the world in different ways than men. They began developing a theory they named "Self-in-Relation" in an attempt to capture some of the ways women operate uniquely in the world. A pivotal premise of this theory is that women's self-esteem depends upon our ability to make and maintain healthy relationships. Men and women may be similar as infants but early on our socialization process takes us in clearly different directions. Men are encouraged to move towards independence, autonomy and self-actualization. Women, however, are guided towards establishing relationships and nurturing them.

Male self-esteem revolves around work and the ability to be autonomous and to succeed in the world. For women, self-esteem is more internally directed. It is clearly tied to the connections we have with others. Our partners, children, family members, friends and acquaintances all become woven into the fabric of our daily emotional lives. When something is "not right" with any of these relationships, our self-esteem suffers. We blame ourselves for the problems and this can lead us to feeling out of control in general and quickly out of control around food. In Part II, we will look at the links between our fears of losing relationships and the ways we hold in thoughts and feelings to maintain the illusion of "good" relationships. *For us to thrive in relationships, grow through them and not run to food when we fear they are threatened, we need to behave assertively, honestly, clearly and in an open-hearted way.* We will revisit this issue later on.

MEET YOUR SUB-SELVES

A number of years ago I was introduced to the concept of *"sub-selves."* Each sub-self has a particular voice and speaks to us at different times throughout the day. They are always with us. I use the idea of sub-selves frequently in my own life and have shared it with clients. Many find it a useful tool in overcoming self-defeating behaviors and it can help you to stop the self-destructive behavior of compulsive eating.

Think of yourself as having many parts or sub-selves. For example, one part we each have is the Adult, who operates in the reality of the moment. We hear our Adult voice when we are thinking things through and making good choices. Our Adult helps us to make sense of the world and our experience in a rational way. This part of us helps us to make mature decisions and to act in ways we feel proud of. Our Adult voice can be useful to bring us back to reality when we get caught up in negative thoughts and feelings. For example, if you have eaten something you wish you had not eaten, like a piece of cake, and you begin beating yourself up about it, you can summon your Adult voice to speak. You do this by saying to yourself, "Reality is, I ate a piece of cake and now I don't feel good about having done so. Reality is, I can learn from this experience. I am noticing that the cake only gave me a brief moment of pleasure. Reality is, I am paying more attention these days to the thoughts and feelings I experience after I eat sweet foods and this awareness is helping me to make important changes. Reality is, I am not perfect and I can choose not to finish eating the rest of the cake (at least most of the time). Reality is being perfect is an unobtainable goal and I am beginning to be more realistic about myself and my behavior." This is a brief example of how your Adult can help you to stop self-destructive patterns and to develop healthier ways to behave. She always begins with the words "Reality is..." and she can ground you in the reality of present time. This helps break your self-destructive thought patterns and helps you to focus your energy in a healthier direction.

Another part each of us entertains at times is our Critical Parent. This is the part of each of us that reminds us of all the things we are doing wrong or of all of our shortcomings. This part can interfere with us in many ways. It can, if we allow it, sap our confidence, lower our self-esteem and plunge us into a negative place. I notice that the Critical Parent is a loud and persistent voice for many women I have worked with. The Critical Parent inside says things like, "Well, you really messed up that time," or "You'll never get it right," or "You'll never be good enough." The message is generally negative, usually not helpful and can keep you beating yourself up.

The cycle goes something like this: I eat chocolate. I feel bad. I criticize myself. I feel worse. I eat more chocolate. Does this sound familiar? You can use your adult to stop this negative cycle by saying something like this: "Reality is I ate chocolate and I notice that I don't feel good physically or emotionally after having done so. Rather than beating myself up about it however, I will just notice how I feel and ask myself what I can learn from this experience. Reality is, I am not perfect and no one else is either. Today I chose to eat chocolate. Reality is I am working towards making different, healthier, more self-loving choices. Reality is I don't have to allow the fact that I ate chocolate to ruin the rest of my day. I choose to move on now. I can bring my focus into present time and let go of what I did in the past."

There are other parts who interact with our Adult and Critical Parent. We have, for example, a Brat who always wants her own way ("Give me that ice cream!"), and a Victim who feels powerless and helpless ("I just can't possibly do anything to help myself or to change!" This is usually spoken in a whining voice.) We also have a Nurturing Parent voice that soothes and comforts us. This is the voice of self-love and appreciation. This is the part of ourselves that most of us listen to far too seldom. This is the voice that we use when we care for a child, for example. We use it when we tell a child that we love them, that they are safe with us, that we will never hurt them. This is a very important voice for us to listen to so we can deliver similar soothing, loving messages to ourselves. We all need to hear them and we seldom get them from outside of ourselves.

When you're having a hard time, treat yourself as you would treat a tiny, hurting child. Nurture yourself. Speak to yourself with patience, kindness and love. Hug yourself then look into your own eyes in a mirror and tell yourself that you will always be there for yourself. Then finish by smiling at your reflection and saying "I love you" to yourself. Try this even if you aren't feeling quite lovable at the time. It is a very powerful and healing exercise.

Now I would like to introduce you to a cunning and crafty part we each have whose "job" it is to undo all of our best intentions. This is the part of us that leads us into bingeing behavior—a strong and active part of most of us. This part is labeled the Saboteur. For the purposes of this book, however, I have renamed her the Chew. The Chew is an unwelcome guest and we often are not even aware of her presence. She is capable of sneaking up on us and, first thing we know, we are doing things that we know are harmful to us. Our Chew can fool us into thinking we are on the right track when, in fact, we may be headed in a self-destructive direction. Let me give you an example. You are at a party and surrounded by foods that are full of sugars and fats. You know that if you eat them you are likely to feel out of control, unhappy with your choice, bloated, etc., but your Chew says, "Go on, have some fun. Eat that sugar and fat. You deserve to enjoy yourself, etc." Instead of sitting down and thinking your options through, you listen to your Chew and eat all you want. Later, you are angry with yourself and feel guilty and negative. Your Chew has won again! She has convinced you to work against your best interest. It is wise to pay close attention to her crafty, sabotaging messages so you will be able to recognize them and resist them. In the second half of this book, we will look at ways to recognize when our Chews are slipping their compelling, evil messages into our heads and I will offer suggestions to help you to send your Chew on her way.

We each have an entire cast of sub-selves inside who compete for our attention and our behavior is influenced by which voice we are listening to at the time. Knowing they are there is a start to understanding yourself, not only regarding your food behaviors but all behaviors you perform. Pay attention to the voices inside of you and the messages they are sending you. As you understand your sub-selves and how they all work together, you will have more power to stay in control of your behaviors. When we don't understand that there are many parts of us that operate at different times, our behavior seems mysterious and beyond our control. We don't think we can do anything to change our course and our Victim (a good friend of our Chew) takes over. We make destructive choices over and over again. We feel bad about ourselves and our Critical Parent (another good friend of our Chew) reminds us of just how bad we really are. It is a cycle. The negative messages and feelings of helplessness go on and on. *We can never rid ourselves of these troublesome voices. It is part of our humanness to have them. We can, however, learn ways to recognize those voices quickly and replace their negative messages with positive ones. We can talk to ourselves in our Adult voice, break self-destructive cycles and resume control.*

BLACK AND WHITE THINKING

It appears to me that most of us who grew up in families that were "dysfunctional" in some way (and that covers just about everybody) learned to think and act in black and white ways a good deal of the time. Food is good or bad. We are either restricting food or binge-ing. Feelings are happy or sad. We love someone completely or not at all. The list of examples is endless. Thinking in dichotomies may appear to make life easier. We can label something as positive or neg-ative and that is the end of that. The world, however is *not* black and white—it is complex and rich and not simple.

I notice that clients report they have either been "good" (mean-ing they have been true to their diet) or "bad" (meaning they have not been faithful to their eating plan and have been overeating). This kind of thinking can get us into a lot of trouble. Because it is impossible to be perfect, we will all have times when we make choices that are not in our best interest. If we then berate ourselves and see ourselves as "bad" we are likely to feel "bad" the rest of the day. (This is one of the many ways our Chew has of getting the upper hand.) If we can instead step back a minute and think about the situation, we can rec-ognize that one choice does not have to ruin the rest of our day. It doesn't even have to affect the next minute.

Instead of reacting to a less than self-loving choice by beating our-selves up and punishing ourselves, we can use each situation to learn more about ourselves. Then we become more understanding of our-selves and we can treat ourselves more gently. We can assure our-selves that one choice is just that—one choice. We may regret that choice, but we can use it as a learning experience and move forward with renewed commitment to make more healthy choices and to treat ourselves and our bodies well as often as we can. Please keep in mind that no one can do exactly the perfect thing for each situation at each and every moment. If we allow ourselves to think in black and white ways, we will stay focused on the errors we make in judgment and keep ourselves stuck in negative patterns.

For example, if each time we eat something that isn't precisely what our eating plan calls for, we tell ourselves we are "all bad" for doing so, we perpetuate a negative belief about ourselves. This will damage our self-esteem, lead us to punish and berate ourselves and set ourselves up to fail again. We reinforce how "bad" we are and later punish ourselves by overeating again. This negative thinking keeps our self-destructive cycle in motion and our self-esteem level low. It is crucial to recognize that there are shades of gray in all of our experiences. Overeating is not "good" or "bad." One choice doesn't make us "good" or "bad." In the above example, reality is (hear your Adult?) that out of all the choices you made today, you made one choice that was not self-loving. You can learn from this experience by noticing how you feel about yourself when you overeat and you can think about ways to make a more self-loving choice next time you are in a similar situation. We need to learn to recognize and appreciate the richness and complexity of our lives and stop black and white thought patterns.

Each day is likely to contain elements that we experience as pleasant and others that are not as pleasurable. We may think that if we experience something unpleasant, something is wrong with us and we need to fix something or change our feelings. We do not. We need only to move through each feeling into the next. There is balance to everything. We are likely to feel many different things every day— happy, sad, angry, delighted, tired, etc. Each day is composed of many events and the various feelings that accompany them. *Black and white thinking stops the flow of our experience and leads us to a stuck and destructive place.* There are many shades of gray to be aware of.

One of the ways we may exhibit black and white thought is in our need to appear perfect at all times to those around us. We may think others will not like or love us if they realize we have flaws. Of course they have flaws as well and would most likely feel closer to us and more comfortable with us if we shared our human frailties with them. If both people in any relationship are honest with each other and share themselves freely, they can relax. They can then feel truly close and connected. We all have this need to feel connected and loved.

Sometimes we fear others will abandon us if we are not perfect. In our efforts to appease them, we may overlook conflicts and issues. We may think and do all sorts of things to try to please others and to win their approval. For example, we may think:

> "If only I am good enough no one will get angry with me or abandon me."
>
> "If I'm perfect, no one will find fault with me."
>
> "If I'm perfect, he/she will love me."
>
> "If I'm perfect, others will look up to me and I will feel safe and satisfied."

This is faulty thinking. We create an illusion of safety when we think in this way. We think behaving perfectly is necessary to keep people near us. This is an illusion. It is a powerful one and difficult to shatter. There are perfect things we can identify (e.g. a perfect moment, a perfect performance by an exceptional artist) but *if we set perfection as our goal, we will be forever frustrated.* Since there is no way to achieve this goal, we will continuously see ourselves as failures.

It is worth taking a few minutes of time to think this through. What is perfection anyway? What does it really mean to be perfect? I think of it as being "flawless, without defect—doing *exactly* the right thing at the right time, *every* time—*never* making a mistake." What does it mean for you? It may mean *never* getting angry or *never* feeling depressed. Maybe it means *never* eating sugar or *never* eating too much of anything. Maybe it means *never* making a mistake or *never* running out of energy. Perhaps it means weighing ninety-eight pounds and having your weight *never* fluctuate. Or maybe it means *never* getting confused or overwhelmed or anxious or feeling out of control in *any* situation. Or it might mean smiling and being pleasant *all the time.* Maybe it means *never* feeling needy or crying. Are any of these likely or possible? *Of course they are not!* That doesn't mean, however that we don't set ourselves up with these impossible goals. When we do, we always fail. Then our Critical Parent voice reminds us loudly of our imperfection and our Chew leads us to the refrigerator.

It is amazing how many women do expect the impossible of themselves. Many times women will admit to me that, although they realize how foolish these expectations sound on an intellectual level, they *do* hold themselves to these standards. As women we don't have these expectations of anyone else, of course, but we often do consider ourselves to be exceptions to the rule. We operate with a double standard. We think we must transcend human error and that we alone should be perfect. We seldom stop to consider how impossibly foolish this idea really is. We have been socialized to think we must be all things to all people and so, to keep others happy, we may give ourselves messages such as:

"I never get angry."
"I never reveal my feelings, unless they are happy ones."
"I never feel down or depressed."
"I never eat too much."

Of course these are unrealistic self-expectations and again supply us with false security. On the surface we may appear happy and peaceful—underneath we may be seething with anger or depressed.

When we are not true to ourselves and expect ourselves to behave as *perfect machines,* we set ourselves up to fail again and again. We overeat. We do this because we have failed again. We may then feel even more ashamed, worthless or frustrated, and punish ourselves further by eating even more. This can go on and on and on. It is a negative, destructive cycle and it is set in motion each time we deny our human frailties and try to do the impossible.

Of course our Chew applauds these actions and urges us to be even more impossibly perfectionistic. Because our Chew is smart she knows that our repeated failures to be perfect assure that her needs to eat ravenously and compulsively will continue to be met. Abandoning black and white thinking, being in the reality of the moment and accepting that no one (not even us) is perfect will help to quiet the insistent voice of your Chew and to calm her down.

Reflections

CHAPTER **IV**

*U*nderstanding the *S*ocial *R*easons for *O*vereating

UNDERSTANDING SELF-IMAGE

OUR self-image is our conception of ourselves. It is not stationary or solid. It is fluid and evolves over time. As we grow and change, the way we view ourselves and present ourselves to the world changes. Most of us grew up being told how to look and act and feel and we developed standards for ourselves and expectations of ourselves based on the messages we received from others—from our families and friends, from institutions such as our schools and churches and from the larger society. These externally imposed messages may not have matched how we truly wanted to be and chances are we didn't look, act and feel the ways we thought we "should." We most likely received messages to be smart, thin and pretty—to be ever-smiling and nurturing of others' needs. Many of us struggled valiantly to fit into the picture of ourselves that others painted for us and we were led to believe that this effort would bring us acceptance, approval and love. What happened instead was that we learned through our struggle that we were not acceptable just as we were.

I remember as a young girl watching friends with straight hair spending hours in agonizing curlers while curly-haired friends bent over their ironing boards to iron and straighten their locks. Short girls were buying high heel shoes while their taller friends searched

63

for flats. Girls who were well-endowed at a young age were dressing to conceal their curves while the flat-chested ones were padding their bras. No one seemed to feel acceptable just as they were. I know I certainly didn't!

The directions we receive from outside of ourselves about how to be in the world shape us as we mature. We want to be the best mothers, partners, spouses, friends, workers, etc. that we can be and so we may continue trying to live up to externally imposed, unrealistic standards and expectations. We may buy bags of makeup and color our hair. We may diet and run miles and miles a day in pursuit of a perfect, thin body. We may cook and clean and care-take others. As discussed in the previous section on black and white thinking, we may continue to pursue the illusive, impossible goal of perfection and to search for the acceptance, love and approval we crave. We will always fall short, however when we try to live up to unrealistic images and our self-image will continue to suffer. The more we try to force ourselves to match an image that is imposed upon us, the less likely we are to be comfortable with ourselves and the more we will see ourselves as failures. This endless effort to match unrealistic, imposed ways of being is at the core of negative self-image. As long as we try to be anything other than who we truly are, our self-esteem will suffer and our self-image will continue to be poor.

We may also have been given specific messages regarding our eating behaviors or body size. Did anyone ever see you eat and say something like: You eat just like fat old aunt Sassy! Or, Wow! What a hippo you're going to be! As we begin to question some of these old messages and to share our feelings and experiences with each other, we empower ourselves to be unique and creative. Our self-esteem level increases and our self-image changes in positive ways. Think about why you really want to stop eating compulsively. Are you truly making this effort for yourself or because you feel compelled by forces outside of yourself? As we challenge and discard the old negative messages we have been receiving all of our lives, we claim the right to be truly ourselves—to be authentic, genuine. Our self-love grows. Self-esteem and self-image improve and we are less likely to become victims of our Chews.

As we pass through the years, we receive different messages about how to be acceptable in our world. As we grow older, we may be told to move aside and let others lead the way. Aging does not mean being feeble or foolish. It does not mean being passive and quietly retreating from the action of the world. It does not mean deferring to others nor does it mean being unattractive or less than vibrant. As wise women (of any age), our self-image does not have to depend upon fulfilling society's expectations. No matter what our chronological age, we can each claim our place as wise women who have much beauty, creativity, energy and love to share.

As we progress from being outer-directed to being inner-directed we build confidence and acquire the wisdom that accompanies life experience. We no longer have to search outside of ourselves to find out how to look and feel and act. We can go within and choose what fits for us at that time. Perhaps later we may feel differently and choose another way to look and act. What matters is that we follow our hearts and be ourselves—ever growing, ever changing—always a wonderful work in progress!

We can start right now following our inner guidance. We can toss out all the old messages and replace them with loving, positive ones. We can give these freely to ourselves. We can celebrate our lively spirits and radiate joy. We can give ourselves the nurturance, love and respect we crave. We don't need to wait for others to give us good feelings. We can connect with each other, validate each other's experience, support each other's growth and have fun together. As we blossom, our self-esteem will improve, our self-image will become more and more positive and we will be less likely to allow our Chew to have the upper hand.

THE OBSESSION

Dieting is an obsession in our culture and the diet industry is a multi-billion dollar enterprise. We are bombarded with messages to be thin and to try fad diet products, diet pills, and wraps that promise to "melt off pounds" while we do nothing. There are liquids that promise to provide balanced nutrition and to help us drop pounds at the same time. There are diet wafers, soft drinks and candies that promise to satisfy our needs while our inches disappear. There is always a new scheme coming along—some kind of product linked to some kind of magical promise. We all know on some level that these do not work. The idea of a quick solution to such a painful problem is alluring, however, and difficult to pass up. Instead of staying with our reasoning selves, we slide into denial and we buy yet another gimmick in a desperate attempt to end our battle with weight once and for all. As many of us know through painful experience, this ends in failure and our self-esteem suffers yet another blow.

The diet industry also makes money in separate but connected ways. It profits from the laxatives and diuretics many women abuse in fruitless and often dangerous attempts to control weight. The industry promotes cosmetics and exercise equipment with promises to us that we will look younger, slimmer, more attractive, etc. Have you ever noticed how happy, relaxed and slim the models on television appear as they demonstrate how to exercise on your new piece of equipment? They appear to be having a wonderful time. Have you ever noticed how you *don't* feel that way when you get on that same equipment at home and begin to breathe harder and to sweat? How many pieces of exercise equipment have you bought and not used for long?

We are urged to color our hair, hide our wrinkles, and cram our bulges into tight clothing until we can barely breathe. We cannot pass a magazine rack without being assaulted by messages that our bodies are not okay. Virtually every issue of any magazine written for women, will contain some kind of article on how to become younger, more beautiful, more slender, more something. *The message is clear. We are never all right just as we are.*

As with any industry, the diet industry only continues to grow if their products *remain in demand.* Have you ever thought about that? If diet products really *did* work, the industry would put itself out of business. Why then are millions of women buying more and more diet products? If diet products *work* and we become thin using them, then why do we need more and more of them? Why do more and more weight loss groups and organizations form? Why? These are important questions to think about. The more informed you are, the more you will be able to steer clear of false promises. You will save money, but, more importantly, you will protect yourself from further disappointment and shame.

KEEPING OURSELVES DISTRACTED

By focusing on our weight and our appearance and by numbing our feelings with food, we keep our minds distracted. Millions of women are constantly preoccupied with thoughts of food, their bodies and their weight and I have wondered, "What would all these women be thinking about if their minds and their energy were not occupied worrying about what they eat and how they look?" A good question, I think. Would women be more likely to set and achieve goals, to empower themselves in some way, to assume more prominent roles in our society? Would there be more programs created designed to eliminate injustices in the world? Would there be less domestic violence? I wonder. What do you suppose you would be thinking about if not food and your weight?

Take a few minutes to consider this question. Close your eyes. Slowly take a few very deep breaths and think about how often you are focused on your eating behavior and your appearance. Think about what things you would rather expend your energy thinking about. Note any thoughts that pass through your mind. Notice any areas of interest or conflict that emerge. Ask yourself what you can do to develop one of those interests or to resolve one conflict. Sit with these thoughts for a few moments. When you feel finished, you can open your eyes and return to the book. What is important here is not that you discovered a long list of interests to pursue or conflicted situations to remedy. What is helpful is that you took time to go inside of yourself and to notice your thought process. You may not have noticed any interests or conflicts emerging. That is fine. The exercise is merely to remind you that there are other things in life besides food and appearance to occupy your mind. Use this exercise every so often to take a look at your priorities. If you are consumed (no pun intended) with thoughts of food and your appearance, this exercise can help you to put those worrisome thoughts into perspective.

RUSHING TO GET "THERE"

This is a fast paced world and most of us live our lives racing along. We seem to think we are going to get somewhere and when we do, we will be able to stop and rest. Where exactly is it that we think we will get to? What will have to happen for us to have finally arrived "there?" Does "there" mean being at a certain career level or seeing a particular number appear when we step onto the scale? Does "there" mean having a certain kind of relationship or car or amount of money? Are we ever content just to be who we are, where we are or what we are? Are we ever happy with what we have, what we look like, what we do? As you have done in previous sections, close your eyes, breathe slowly and take some time to think about yourself and these questions.

I notice that women who come to talk with me about their struggles with food and weight most often are keeping themselves so busy that these basic questions have never entered their minds. They think that there is some miracle place that they will get to at some point and all their worry and stress will dissolve. They think there will come a time when they will no longer have difficult issues to confront or problems to solve. This will *not* happen. What does happen, for example, when you lose an amount of weight? Do you sit back and enjoy your new body size? Do you feel relaxed and proud of yourself? Is the struggle really over? No, not usually. Instead you fear that you will regain every pound and more. You may even become more anxious and stressed. There is *never* a time when you can relax and say "It's over." When you get *there,* there is no *there* there! So rushing towards an unattainable goal gets us nowhere. I suggest you spend some time thinking about this and rethinking your priorities.

Think about why you want to stop eating compulsively at this particular time. You will be ever frustrated and discontented with yourself, your life and your weight if you fail to appreciate yourself and your situation in present time. We spend most of our time living in the past or future. It is challenging to stay in the present. What we have in reality is only the present moment to enjoy. We are always thinking of things we did or didn't do in the past or worrying about what we will or won't do or have in the future. We miss the present moment and our lives go by without our even being aware of the passage of time. We remain out of touch with ourselves this way. Staying in the present helps us appreciate our experiences and ourselves. Obsessing about the past or future keeps us disconnected from ourselves and our experience. This disconnection keeps us anxious and unhappy and our Chew appreciates that.

Instead of focusing on what you *don't* have yet, think about what you *do* have. This requires an attitude adjustment and is difficult for most of us. To appreciate who we are and where we are, we have to slow down and pay attention. This is not easy in our fast-paced world. I urge you to take quiet time to be alone. Take time out to breathe and think and to be by yourself *every single day.* Often women tell me that it is impossible for them to find time for themselves. I respond by asking them to think about their priorities. Making time means putting your own needs first and making yourself your absolute top priority. This is not just important. *This is essential.* If you are to lose weight and feel comfortable in your body and in your life situation, you will have to slow down and nurture yourself. If you do not do this, you will remain out of touch with yourself and you will continue to eat to submerge feelings of resentment, discontent and frustration. If you spend your life rushing to get from here to *there,* there will just be another *there* to get to. Think about it. Where are you trying to get to in such a hurry? What do you want to accomplish for yourself in this lifetime? *Where are you on your list of priorities? Are you even on the list? If not, perhaps it's time to put yourself and your needs at the very top of your list!*

GENDER IN SOCIETY

Could it be that the messages we receive in this culture are designed to keep us feeling inferior, powerless, and isolated? Do they prevent us from developing our talents? . . . following our dreams? . . . facing conflicts in our lives? If so, it makes sense to distract ourselves to avoid facing the reality of our positions in society. Let's consider for a moment what we are told from girlhood on in our development. As infants, girls have historically been valued less than boys. When I was told that my first born was a male, I felt proud that I had given birth to the heir of the family name. He was important and superior somehow. I felt a vague sense of vicarious importance through him. Why? I didn't question my reaction then but I do now. And now I ask, why are males more highly valued? Why are only girl children offered for adoption from China? Why not boys? Girls are not prized in the same way boys are. Why? What's going on here? Why aren't little girls treated in the same way their brothers are? On their recording *City Down,* Casselberry-DuPree sing a song entitled *"Did Jesus Have A Baby Sister?"* and speculate in their lyrics about whether we would have heard of her if he had. What do you think?

As little girls we learned partly through fairy tales and approved play. We listened to stories such as Snow White, Cinderella and Sleeping Beauty. Many of us lived for the day when Prince Charming's kiss would awaken us (often from an "evil" mother figure) and he would lift us lovingly, with adoration in his sparkling eyes, onto his white horse to gallop blissfully toward some destiny known as "happily ever after." His kiss would literally breathe life into us. No one went on to tell us that we wouldn't all marry "princes." Even though we may have observed how hard our mothers worked to provide for our family, these stories offered us hope that our lives would magically be different. No one told us that our marital contract would include cleaning toilets, making sure our husband had clean clothes every day and hot meals on the table. No one ever mentioned that this spouse might not make enough money on his own to support us and that we might need to work in a factory or put in long, exhausting hours as a waitress to make ends meet. No one ever said our partner might not always shower love and wealth upon us. Did anyone ever tell you these things? No one told me.

We received many different messages as we watched these apparently innocent fairy tales. If we examine these messages, we discover that all the heroines are fair-skinned (so we should be—what a negative message to women of color), petite (so we should be tiny if we expect Prince Charming to choose us), and distrusting of other women (remember it was a female figure who poisoned Snow White, who mistreated Cinderella and who plotted to destroy Sleeping Beauty). We also find that all three heroines are passive and dependent upon the attention of a male to awaken their senses and to literally breathe life into them (so we should be passive and dependent as well). These were the role models for many of us.

How do you suppose we were affected as we listened to these stories or watched these movies with rapt attention? Did many or most of us absorb the message that we are inferior? Did some of us make a decision back then to emulate these heroines—to be tiny, pale, passive? Did we also learn to distrust the females in our lives—our mothers, our sisters, our friends? What was the effect of these pale, thin images on each of us? How did young women-of-color respond to all this, or girls with medium or larger body types, or girls who preferred girls to boys as confidants or objects of their affection?

I would mention here that there are books being created today for children that challenge old stereotypes for both boys and girls. I would urge you to examine and purchase these not only for the little children in your life but also for yourself. We each have a little child inside who can and will respond when we re-think some of the old assumptions we made as children. We can challenge old beliefs and nurture ourselves and our children at the same time. When I read to my grandchildren, for example, I am giving attention not only to them but also to myself. I am giving myself some of the attention I craved as a child. This is good—an act of love and healing for myself and for the child on my lap. If you are blessed with small children in your life spend time with them. Read to them. Talk with them. Play games with them. This will be wonderful for them and very helpful for you at the same time. If you don't have children, perhaps you might visit a neighbor or friend with children or volunteer some time in a day care center. Take advantage of any opportunity you can create to enjoy being "child-like" with a child.

THE RELATIONSHIP BETWEEN PRIVILEGE AND GENDER

We learned early in our lives that boys were more important than girls. We learned to be subservient and to conceal our urgings for excitement, autonomy and power. If we secretly dreamed of being pirates or explorers, we may have privately wondered if something was wrong with us for having such bold or ambitious thoughts. We saw our selection by "the prince" and our journey to "happily ever after" as a goal we were supposed to strive for and many of us abandoned our secret dreams because we felt forced to fit into society's expectations of us. Everyone wants approval. To get it we may have had to adjust ourselves to the norms of society while privately yearning for more challenging options or life choices.

When I was a girl, I was basically offered three careers to choose from. I could be a nurse, a teacher or a secretary. Period. It didn't matter that none of these excited me. I was told my career choice wasn't important anyway because I only needed "something to fall back on in case my husband, prince charming himself (who would of course be supporting me), died." This seems ridiculous in retrospect but it does accurately reflect the common thinking of that time. I feel excited now when I hear a little girl assert that she plans to be a doctor or an astronaut and even more excited and hopeful when I hear her dreams supported by her parents and teachers. Perhaps these girls will escape the anxiety that manifests when choices and freedom to grow are denied. Perhaps eating concerns won't be as prominent for them as they focus their attention on their goals instead of their size. Maybe their Chews will be more tame.

Messages concerning the *devaluing* of women come to us through all our societal institutions, not just through play and fairy tales. In government we continue to be severely underrepresented. In the workplace women are still not paid fairly. Religious structures often discriminate against women by assigning males to carry out the most valued roles and women to handle the less glamorous and unimportant ones. As a woman becomes aware in our patriarchal society, she cannot help but notice that her options are limited in some important ways by her gender. Women in the workforce, to be respected as much as a male peer, must be twice as effective and when women and men behave in the same ways, men are viewed as assertive and productive while women are seen as aggressive and domineering. Is it any wonder that girls who are bright and motivated may become anxious as they mature and realize what limited choices they have?

What does a girl see as her opportunity for a successful, rich and rewarding life? Does she become frustrated, fearful and anxious? And, if so, where does the inevitable anxiety lead her? If she seeks equality and is prevented from experiencing it, where does she turn for consolation? Does she turn to chocolate cake or to cookies? Does she begin a pattern of bingeing and/or withholding food? Does she choose drugs, alcohol, gambling, sex, or some other self-destructive behavior to numb her feelings? As you remember those formative years in your own life, can you recall having an experience like this? What did you see then as opportunities? What were your options? If the prospects were nonexistent, how did you cope with your feelings about that? Did you medicate and calm yourself by overeating even then?

LIMITED OPTIONS

Women I have counseled report that when they entered adolescence and later approached adulthood, they frequently found themselves with difficult choices to make. Some were unable to find any inspiring role models. The options were few. On the one hand, they could marry, raise a family and perhaps work in a non-fulfilling setting (as they may have seen their mothers do) or they could choose an altogether different path and enter into a career as their priority. Either choice carried with it anxiety-producing drawbacks.

If a young woman chose to be like her mother, she may have chosen that role joyously and consciously. She may have genuinely felt fulfilled in her position as wife and mother. She may have found she gained her mother's approval but had a less than rewarding or challenging life. If she chose a career over raising a family, she may have found herself in a rewarding professional situation but she may have damaged her bond with her mother in the process. She may have incurred her mother's disapproval or envy. Because the mother/daughter relationship carries within it so much power, this dilemma is a very serious one for many women. Making frightening choices, risking failure, facing your mother's anger or risking the possible loss of a relationship causes anxiety. Our anxiety can be a catalyst for many of the self-destructive behaviors we use to numb our feelings, or to distract or punish ourselves.

Women are constantly faced with the choice to adhere to gender roles as prescribed by our culture or to challenge those roles and to perform in new ways. Whenever a woman steps out of the main stream in any way she risks disapproval. If she is too passive or considered overly aggressive, she is discounted. If she is too short, too old or too heavy, she is often looked down upon. If a woman is of color or lesbian or bisexual, her diversity is not celebrated. This is a society that does not generally value or celebrate difference of any kind. It is also a society that does not generally value or appreciate women.

For a woman to fit nicely into our society's ideal picture, she must be young, white, heterosexual, tall, and thin. She must be smiling, calm and understanding at least 95% of the time. She must be willing to put others' needs ahead of her own at all times and be content with less than equal opportunities and wages. This ideal woman must be smart, but not too smart. She must be active, but not too active, and passive, but not too passive. She must be able to take care of herself but not appear to be too independent. Is it any wonder that women are so often anxious and confused? We are asked to be all and to be nothing. The messages we receive are "crazy-making," impossible to live up to and harmful to us as women.

We cannot be bombarded with messages from society that we are unimportant and feel good about ourselves. The two do not go together. If our culture sets impossible ideals for us, then our culture sets us up to fail. If we try to live up to the images we are presented with, then we set ourselves up to fail as well. If we feel like failures, we will either stop eating altogether or feel unable to control our overeating as a result. Our Chew will thrive and we will continue to make unhealthy choices, such as consuming huge amounts of food, to quiet these confused, frustrating and anxious feelings.

Reflections

CHAPTER V

Understanding the Spiritual Reasons for Overeating

A LOOK AT OUR REAL NEEDS

IN my experience, women who don't care about themselves or their lives do not come through my door struggling with food control issues. On the contrary, women who seek my services are generally intelligent, motivated, creative, and perfectionistic. For the most part, women who ask for help are energetic and resourceful, but much of their energy is tied up obsessing about food or weight. Because of their eating habits, their physical energy is often low and because of their poor self-esteem, their emotional energy is also affected. These women frequently report a sense of being alone in their struggle. As I have said before, we all have a strong need for connection—to feel loved, accepted, and cared about. Without the presence of these feelings, at least some of the time, life's battles quickly become overwhelming and the task of treating ourselves with compassion, respect and nurturance seems impossible. We cannot count on others to give us these good feelings. We must learn to give them to ourselves by finding the love, connection and energy we have deep inside.

I am convinced that within each of us there exists a center where we love ourselves, and harbor the desire to grow and to be creative. Our creativity may shine when we are writing, drawing, cooking, gardening, knitting or listening to a friend, for example. As women we want to reach out, to stretch ourselves beyond our familiar, daily routines but we often feel afraid or stuck. Being obsessed with body size and food keeps our energy tied up and this can provide us with an illusion of safety. We don't have to confront our fears and move forward if we focus on winning this war we are raging against our bodies. Being obsessed with food is like being in a prison where we are both the jailer and the jailed. To break out of our self-imposed prisons we need to develop our spiritual selves. This is a vital part of the process of freeing ourselves to grow and to develop to our greatest potential.

We can understand the reasons why we have developed unhealthy eating habits. We can become experts on nutrition and learn better ways to manage our stress. We can look at the ways society has encouraged our passivity and dependency and we can strategize about ways to cope within our daily lives and make constructive changes. Without some element of spirituality, however, we are unlikely to win our battle for food control or to attain a feeling of peace in our lives. We need to know there is more to life than struggle. We must learn to go within to find meaning.

When I first began to think about the essential part that spirituality plays in women's lives and wanted to begin discussing this with my clients, I was fearful that I might offend a woman if she did not hold a particularly spiritual view of herself or her world. What a delightful surprise when I found, without exception, that every client I talked with was receptive to the idea of exploring and developing her "inner-self" or her "spirit." Instinctively we all seem to know we are spiritual beings. You may never have had the time or encouragement to think about yourself in this way, however. Doing so now can help you to feel less alone, less frightened. If you are in touch with your spiritual self, you will be able to journey within yourself to find the comfort and love you need at any time.

UNDERSTANDING SPIRITUALITY

Many of us have a hard time defining spirituality for ourselves. Let me take a moment here to clarify that when I speak of spirituality, I am not referring to religion. Most of us were raised within an organized religion. Many of us chose to stop attending to that religion when we became adults. I am not suggesting a return to religious practice, although for some that may be helpful. I am suggesting that you develop the ability to turn inward and listen to your own voice—that voice which is heard (faintly at first) deep within your core self. To hear this voice, however, you must be still and many of us have a hard time finding that stillness.

In December of 1995, a conference called *Spirituality and Healing* was cosponsored by Harvard Medical School and The Mind/Body Institute of the Deaconess Hospital in Boston, Massachusetts. Spirituality was defined at this assembly as "the belief that we all have meaning and purpose in life and that on a profound level we are all connected." This may ring true for many of us. However, each of us is unique and thus our perceptions of spirit are as varied as we are. In her beautiful book of daily meditations, *The Language of Letting Go*, Melody Beattie states, "We're learning to take care of our emotions, our mind and our physical needs. We're learning to change our behaviors. But we're also learning to take care of our spirit, *our soul*, because that is where all true change begins."

You chose this book because you wish to make changes. To do so permanently, you must first learn about yourself as a spiritual being and heal your spirit as Ms. Beattie suggests. What is spirit? When are we in touch with our spirit? We may feel "spirit" when we view a breathtaking sunset or watch a baby take his or her first step. We may feel "spiritual" when we kiss a child goodnight or pat an animal or read a beautiful poem. Being spiritual means being alive and in touch with yourself and your life in some way. It can mean dancing with joy or singing. It can mean crying cleansing tears or raking leaves. It means many different things to each of us because no two of us are the same. It also means appreciating that you are special and unique.

When I think of my own spirituality, I think of being aware of myself and my connection to all other beings on this planet. My spiritual self strives to be unconditionally loving and accepting of myself and others and to be forgiving as well. This is, of course, not possible all of the time. When I am in touch with my spirit, I am grateful for my life and feel a reverence for all living things. Through this awareness of myself as connected to some universal source, I feel empowered to take actions on my own behalf and to take responsibility for myself. I find peace and comfort in my spiritual practice, through prayer and meditation and living as mindfully as possible.

At other times, however, I am out of touch with spirit. Then I feel lonely and can easily become depressed and anxious. Food looms in front of me promising relief and my Chew begs for attention. If I re-establish my connection to spirit at that time through meditation or prayer, food once again recedes into the background. If not, a negative cycle begins. Life is a process of remembering and forgetting—of connecting and disconnecting. Please note, by the way, *there is no right or wrong way to develop our spiritual selves and there is no way to do it perfectly either. We are all human and it is the human way, remember, not to be perfect.*

THE SPIRITUAL PROCESS

For each of us, the process is one of remembering and forgetting. When we find ourselves tangled up in worry and stress, when we find ourselves thinking of chocolate or potato chips, we feel ashamed and flood with negative feelings. We are reminded by these feelings that we have forgotten something very important. We have forgotten that we are spiritual beings. Realizing this is good. We can choose to listen to this message and make changes or ignore it and fall into old self-destructive habits. We can pay attention and do something to bring ourselves back to a centered place where we can find peace or ignore it and continue eating in a self-destructive way. We can continue *feeding* our negative feelings or stop and choose a more self-loving behavior (e.g. meditate, write in a journal, go for a walk in the country). We can *choose* either course of action. We are not powerless and we become empowered when we give ourselves what we really need: loving energy and quiet time to reflect and reconnect with spirit. Although we may continue to choose chocolate on occasion, we make that choice knowing next time we may make a different, more self-loving one.

If you choose to bring yourself "back to center" you might meditate for twenty minutes or spend a little time writing in your journal. You might paint or put on some music and dance. A half an hour of yoga or Tai Chi works for many women as might a long relaxing bath with candlelight and soft music. Spirituality is different and unique to each of us. It does, however, mean putting aside the distractions of our lives temporarily and going inside to notice the feelings we are having and to listen to what our own voices are telling us. Whether your idea of spirituality includes a concept of some kind of god or not is not what is important. *That you acknowledge the spirit within yourself is what counts.* It means acknowledging yourself as a woman who is special—who is creative and expressive. It means celebrating the life and energy within your own being.

For most of us, the demands that accompany our roles in life keep our minds and bodies otherwise occupied. We are busy, busy, busy making sure everyone else is okay. For many of us, our energy goes out to children, partner or spouse, work, home, pets, extended family, yard work, and on and on. There often seems no end to the concerns which occupy us. How often do most of us set everything aside to tune into our internal state of affairs? When was the last time you actually set aside time to consider your life and your own feelings and needs? When was the last time you *really* paid attention to yourself?

HOW WE IGNORE SPIRIT

Overeating helps to keep us numb and giving ourselves the time and space we deserve to reflect on our emotions and dreams can be difficult for many of us. We may be keeping ourselves outwardly distracted to prevent ourselves from facing our lives, and our feelings about our lives. Keeping "over busy" is akin to overeating. Each serves to keep us superficially content, at least temporarily. We can zip about appearing to be doing well but privately we may know that we are not! We may eat or work ourselves to exhaustion to avoid facing the reality of our situations. In this way we lose ourselves. In this way we ignore our real needs and our spirit suffers. My experience is that as long as we race around like robots and fail to attend to our own feelings and needs, we are likely to substitute food (or excessive work, sex, gambling, alcohol, drugs, etc.) for the satisfaction and contentment we are not experiencing. Most women who seek my services are busily focused outside of themselves in this way.

The more focused you are on outward appearance and seeking approval from the outside, the more difficult it will be for you, at least initially, to journey within. For some of you, the idea of any spiritual connection may be foreign and you may have no idea where to begin. One way to start is just to notice your breath and to sit quietly for a few minutes each day paying attention to your breathing and to any feelings or thoughts that may arise. I am not sure if anyone really understands why sitting quietly in this way often leads to exploration of one's spiritual self but many people report that it does. We are usually so outwardly focused that just being quiet and listening to ourselves breathe can turn our consciousness inward to a peaceful place. We will talk more about some specific ways to do this in the section on *Healing the Spiritual Self* in Part II of this book. For now, just know that *going inside to attend to yourself and your needs is an essential step in the process of letting go of any addiction.* This may seem foreign and even threatening right now, however, as you read on, you will see that it need not be scary to look within yourself and to listen to your heart. Ultimately it can and will liberate you from your prison of compulsive eating. It will definitely help you to *Quiet your Chew.*

Reflections

PART II

WAYS TO HEAL—
HOW TO CHANGE

IN the first half of this book we looked at many of the reasons we may have begun to eat compulsively in the first place. We have examined the causes holistically—that is, considering the physical, emotional, social and spiritual factors that have contributed to the development of our self-destructive behavior. Now in Part II, we move in a different direction and shift the focus from cause to curative action. We move from realizing why behaviors and patterns were established in the first place to examining ways to change these self-destructive behaviors and to break these old patterns. First we look at changes we can make to take better care of ourselves physically and then move on to consider changes we can make emotionally, socially and spiritually.

As you progress through each section, I encourage you to note changes that you think would be particularly helpful for you to make in each of these areas of your life. Each of us is different and so there is no one way to work on these issues. First think of just your physical body and see if you can pinpoint some concrete ways to help yourself become healthier and stronger. The section entitled *Healing the Physical Self* will have lots of suggestions for you. Read through this section to see what changes seem comfortable and possible. Remember, you can't change everything at once, so see if there are one or two ideas that capture your attention and implement those.

Each change you make is one more step away from your old pattern of eating compulsively.

Next, read through the section entitled *Healing your Emotional Self* to discover ways you can make changes in that area. Think of your emotional self and of how you would like to help yourself feel better. Likewise, consider your social and spiritual experiences and consider making changes in these parts of your life as well. It is useful to look at the pieces in this way and, by doing so a plan for change will gradually emerge from the readings. When you have had a chance to think about each of these areas separately, we will go on to part III and begin tying it all together. By the conclusion of this book you will have made a clear, flexible, reasonable plan for yourself which you can follow to improve your relationship with yourself, to stop your compulsive, self-punishing behavior, and to finally *Tame your Chew.*

CHAPTER **VI**

*M*oving from *P*ast into *F*uture

HOW YOU GOT HERE

B
Y reading Part I, you have already taken significant first steps towards changing your compulsive behavior. As you are reading this book, you are gaining a clearer understanding of your relationships with food, with your body, with your feelings and with your spirit and you are learning how societal messages have impacted upon you. As you are educating yourself, you are preparing to move in a healthier direction. You are doing the research necessary for making important, permanent changes in your life. You have begun to understand where some of your self-destructive attitudes and behaviors came from and to recognize many of the ways you have been pressured to diet and to fit into a mold. Armed with this knowledge, you are ready to stop listening to others and to make some different choices. It is time to listen to your own voice.

Food has served some very important purposes for you. As you learn more about this, food no longer serves as an effective way to cope with life's challenges and the feelings that go along with them. Recognizing the negative messages you got from family, society, peers, religion, government, the media, and others about your body and body size helps you to challenge these messages. Realizing that you were expected to please others, to earn their approval as a way of feeling good about yourself, is also crucial knowledge. Knowing this frees you to find other ways to feel good about yourself. Likewise, knowing that the pressure to conform had much to do with your choice to abuse yourself with food helps you to end this self-abuse. All of this knowledge is powerful and will support you in finding and making more self-loving choices.

By realizing how you got here you move automatically into a new place. Please appreciate that you did not create the environment you grew up in. You have been reacting to physical, emotional and social cues and you have been using inappropriate eating behaviors to take care of yourself. You have not been responsible for your self-destructive behaviors in the past. Your overeating has been, instead, a result of all the forces around you and within you. Yes, you did pick up the food and put it into your mouth but it would have been difficult not to do so. You did not have the understanding and the tools necessary for resisting your powerful urges to binge.

Your overeating most likely began as a way of protecting yourself from painful feelings. As a child you had no way to defend yourself or to speak up when people treated you unfairly. You learned that food could "take the edge off" when you were hurt or angry or anxious and you most likely experienced these painful feelings at times because you were bombarded with negative, hurtful messages. At that time, you could not understand the impact of these messages upon you. You chose food to cope with the confusion and pain that you experienced as a result. As you know, this has not worked. Food is not an effective way to cope with difficulties. As we will see, there are better, less painful ways to handle your experiences and feelings and more productive ways to meet life's challenges.

TAKING RESPONSIBILITY

Now that you understand your past, you can prepare to take full responsibility in the present. Taking responsibility day by day, moment by moment, will insure that you continue to do so in the future. In Part II of this book, I will offer practical advice and methods to free you from the past and to change self-destructive behaviors on physical, emotional, social and spiritual levels. Remember, each of us is different, so what seems useful to you may not carry the same importance for another. As you read, please sift out what sounds helpful *for you*. Listen to your inner voice for guidance and let yourself be open to experimenting with new behaviors as you go along.

Taking responsibility for yourself means choosing areas in which you would like to make changes, devising strategies for making these changes and then implementing the strategies you have chosen. After thinking about and targeting ways you can start making changes in each area that we cover, we will move on to the final section of the book entitled *"Summing it all up."* Here you put together a long-term plan for yourself. This will enable you to take responsibility for yourself and to manage your compulsive eating behavior. We will explore some general concepts that will help you plan effective strategies for making powerful changes in the way you view food and your body. You will see that being free from compulsive eating means making changes in your attitudes about yourself and in the ways you approach and live your life.

Although the idea of making such powerful changes may seem overwhelming, it can be done when approached in this way. We will look at how to do this one moment, one step, one day at a time. No significant changes happen over night and no one can do anything perfectly. So try not to think in terms of changing such difficult behavior as an event that will occur and then be over. Instead think of ending your compulsive eating behavior as a process that will continue over time. You make some changes. You experiment. You review and revise your plan as you grow. You make new changes. You have times that are easy, others that are more challenging. *You make a plan, revise it and revise it again. But you are always learning, always changing and always getting closer to yourself.* In this way, you manage your compulsive eating behavior and your Chew will lay dormant more often than not.

Reflections

CHAPTER VII

*H*ealing the *P*hysical *S*elf

DEVELOPING BODY AWARENESS AND FLEXIBILITY

A S mentioned earlier, many women begin to *lose touch* with their bodies as they go through adolescence and enter adulthood. This loss of awareness almost universally happens for women who eat compulsively. Moving our bodies is necessary if our bodies are to perform efficiently. We need to exercise our hearts with aerobic exercise regularly to stimulate our respiratory and circulatory systems. We must do this to oxygenate our blood and to assure that this fresh blood supply reaches all areas of our body. We need to nurture ourselves with exercise, fresh air and sunshine to be fully alive and healthy.

If we are to take the best care of our bodies, we must develop an attitude of *appreciation* towards them; but we cannot appreciate our bodies if we are out of touch with them. We must take necessary actions to reconnect with our bodies. Only then will we be in a position to befriend and care for them. One way to begin this process is to *move*. For many of us, our entrance into adulthood may have marked a time when we stopped using our body to play and have fun and began using it for more adult matters such as giving birth, sitting at our job or watching television. Have you ever watched a small child delight in discovering what his or her body can do? Can you recall ever feeling really free in your own body—just running or hopping or jumping for the fun of it? For many of us it is hard to stay in touch with the fun. Moving has become synonymous with exercise which translates into "work"—not play!

About ten years ago, I ran faithfully every morning. Sunrise was my favorite time. I would watch the colors as the sun poked itself up into the sky and I would chatter with the early morning squirrels. This was *my* time (my kids were still sound asleep in bed) and I loved the feelings I had as I jumped over puddles and kicked little stones along my path. If something interested me, I would stop to examine it more closely and if I felt tired, I would slow down and walk. Sometimes, before I went inside, I would sit by the pond near my house for a few minutes to plan my day or just to think about nothing in particular.

Then one day I decided to enter a women's marathon in a near-by town. Things changed. I began to measure my daily miles and to clock my speed. I no longer gave myself the option of slowing down or walking. I could not miss a single day of practice. I was in competition with myself. Every day I pushed myself to run faster and farther. I was training far too strenuously. I was so busy with all this that I didn't even notice that I had *stopped having fun.* To make a long story short, I did run the race and I did finish. I was second to last and would have been last but for one unfortunate contestant who broke her ankle and was technically the last place finisher. Was my effort worthwhile?

I had missed many mornings of sunrises and bird serenades only to find the race grueling and painful! Some people thrive on the thrills of training and competition. Some people manage to train appropriately and enjoy the experience—not I! This was clearly *not* worth the sacrifice for me. I did not win the race. I did, however, learn an important lesson about myself. Having fun and enjoying my body is definitely more important to me than winning any race ever could be. So I ended my short-lived racing career and once again began "playing" at running and getting back in touch with having fun.

Most of us lose our ability to play with movement as we age. We may get too busy to notice *when and how* we stop having fun with our bodies, but we do. I do not mean that all of the women I meet with are entirely unaware of their bodies. They may be exercising and moving but usually they report that the *fun* is gone. As many other Americans these days, they may be aware of feeling uncomfortable with their physical selves. They might exercise, even fanatically, but view the exercise as a *chore* (more "serious adult work"). They may feel large and uncomfortable in their bodies. They may notice that they wheeze when climbing stairs and they may report that they avoid social situations where they will be using their bodies in front of other people, such as dancing, hiking or bicycling. Seldom do women report that they are in touch with the pure joy of moving their bodies.

We are often cautioned to avoid the "harmful" rays of the sun. Harvey and Marilyn Diamond point out in their book, *Fit for Life* that some sunshine is good for us and that some exposure helps with weight loss and detoxification. They caution us not to avoid the sun entirely but not to spend excessive amounts of time in the sunlight either. Andrew Weil, M.D. in his well known books, *Spontaneous Healing and Eight Weeks to Optimum Health* cautions that exposure to sunshine can cause skin cancer. He suggests we protect ourselves when in the sunshine by wearing protective clothing and using sunscreen. He also cautions us against visiting tanning parlors as the rays emanating from the tanning equipment are as dangerous as direct sunlight. Deepak Chopra, M.D. in his book *Perfect Weight* reminds us that the sun is the source of all life and that by feeling the warmth of the sunshine on our skin we are putting ourselves in contact with the most powerful source of energy on our planet. He suggests, however that we be respectful of the power of this energy and not expose ourselves to "too much of a good thing." Consensus is that experiencing a *small* amount of sunshine may be beneficial. A bit of exposure can improve digestion, help us to lose weight and detoxify our bodies. Some sunshine gives us natural vitamin D and energy and the sun's warmth may improve our mood. Remember, however, to exercise caution. Too much sunlight can be very dangerous.

Appreciation of our bodies comes in a variety of ways. We can allow ourselves to marvel at this "machine" called our body and all that it does for us each moment. We can give ourselves plenty of rest and nutritious food. We can focus on our strength and endurance and our abilities to do many things and we can appreciate the beautiful parts of our bodies. We can also cultivate self-appreciation by beginning to stretch and to move and to rediscover our flexible selves. I recommend activities that encourage you to tune in to your body. Yoga, Tai Chi, and many forms of dance are excellent for this purpose. Other activities, such as swimming, running, walking, bicycling, playing sports, etc. can be helpful when performed consciously and with an attitude of play. When physical activity is undertaken without a playful attitude much of the benefit is lost. What form of movement appeals to you? How will you begin to incorporate some playful exercise into your life?

CHANGING ROBOTIC BEHAVIOR

Begin noticing when, where and how you are eating. Most of us have developed eating patterns over the years that have served us poorly. We may eat while driving, watching television or reading, for example and be totally oblivious to the fact that we are eating at all. I call this "robotic eating." When we fail to notice and appreciate our food, we are acting automatically—like robots. To feel satisfied after eating, we must do more than just fill our stomachs. We must also enjoy the experience we are having. If we attend to our food consciously, we will end our meal satiated physically, emotionally and spiritually. If we perform the ritual of eating without paying to attention to it, we will feel deprived and dissatisfied. We will still hunger for the experience of eating that we completely missed.

I routinely talk with my clients about the experience of "conscious eating" or "eating meditation" and I urge you to try this exercise. First, choose the surroundings in which you will eat your meal and make them as peaceful and relaxing as possible. Use beautiful dishes that give you pleasure. Add candles, flowers, or soft music if you enjoy them. Next, plan your meal. It is important to select and prepare your food with awareness. Choose whole foods that appeal to you and are both nourishing and attractive. Notice their colors, shapes, textures and smells as you prepare them. Take a moment to be thankful for the food you are about to eat and to consider how the eating experience will bring pleasure, nourishment and good health. Next, begin to eat. Do this slowly and with as little distraction as possible. Allow yourself time to relax and to be aware of each bite as you lift it to your mouth. Appreciate the smell, color, texture and taste. Notice how the food feels in your mouth. Chew thoroughly and be aware of the sensations as you swallow. At the end of your meal, take a moment to be thankful for the food you have eaten, for your body and for the health you are promoting. This experience will bring you satisfaction not only physically, but emotionally and spiritually as well. You will have eaten with consciousness and care. You will know that you have given your *whole* self the attention you deserve and you will feel satisfied.

Of course you will not have the time to eat all your meals this slowly and consciously. Do so at least once a week however. In between those times, eat your meals in a relaxed way. Always eat slowly. Do not take a bite of food until you have swallowed the last bite and engage in only pleasant conversation with others. Do not eat if you are not hungry, or if you feel upset, but please do eat whenever you are truly hungry. Eat your main meal of the day at noon and make your dinner a light meal. Do not eat after 6 P.M.

If you must lose weight, try having only liquids one day each week. Choose fresh, organic fruit and vegetable juices, purified water, herbal teas and clear broth for this purpose. If you have any health problems I suggest you consult your medical doctor before beginning any type of fasting program.

Always choose healthy, wholesome fruits and vegetables (organic if possible) and whole grains. Substitute poultry or fish for meat if you do eat meat and try to have at least one or two "meat free" days each week. Avoid caffeine, alcohol, fats, sugar and artificial sweeteners. Experiment with new foods. Try some soy products (you can find an assortment of these in health food stores) and a variety of flavorings and spices. Be creative and express yourself through your meal preparation. If you give your menu planning, food preparation, environment and eating behavior this kind of care and attention, you will feel nurtured. You will be giving yourself the care and attention you deserve and you will feel satisfied.

Many of us spend a good deal of our life performing the tasks of daily living as if we were robots, with little thought or awareness. Many a chocolate bar or bag of chips has disappeared without our realizing we had anything to do with it. A client once told me that she had no idea why she kept gaining weight. She said she felt as if the fat snuck into the room and crept up onto her body while she slept. At the time, she had absolutely no idea of how much she was eating. She felt helpless—like a victim. She had no awareness of the constant snacking she was doing. I asked her to spend one week recording every bit of food that she put into her mouth. This was an eye-opening exercise for her and helped her to develop a consciousness about what she was doing. You might try the same to help yourself become aware of your "robotic" eating times. You need this awareness to stop the automatic, self-destructive behavior.

Do you stop at the candy machine automatically or grab something quick and easy when you are driving? Do you have junk food in the cupboard that you grab when you are reading or watching television? Do you reach for quick snacks instead of preparing meals and do foods seem to disappear from your kitchen or pantry without your knowledge? Put yourself in the role of investigator and identify times when you engage in robotic behavior. By discovering the eating you are doing without awareness, you give yourself the information you need to make different, more self-loving choices. You can then treat yourself more thoughtfully and lovingly and you won't feel like an "out of control" victim of your Chew any longer.

SEEING YOUR WHOLE SELF WITH LOVE

We seldom really see our whole selves. Women often report that they avoid looking in full length mirrors and they hurry past their reflection if it appears by surprise in a store window. Many of us have developed extremely negative images of ourselves and so, even if we do occasionally look at our whole selves, we look with a critical eye. Instead of appreciating the many attractive parts we have, we sometimes see only the negative. Our eyes may gravitate to the thickness of our hips, the roundness of our bellies or our double chins instead of seeing the whole picture. We focus on the parts we don't like and fail to notice the beautiful ones. This has a powerful effect. Seeing ourselves with such disapproval (sometimes hatred?) has a powerful negative effect. If we see isolated parts of ourselves and feel disgusted or angry, we miss any opportunity to feel good about ourselves as a whole.

No one has the perfect physical body. Even models who appear in glamour magazines have their photos touched up before publication. Blemishes and imperfections disappear. Most women fail to measure up to today's unrealistic beauty standards. Please know that you are not alone. All of us have parts of ourselves that we wish were somehow different. Part of the work of letting go of compulsive eating is to accept ourselves as we are and to integrate all the parts of ourselves into a whole being—a whole being whom we can grow to appreciate and to love.

This acceptance of our whole self does not come overnight. It is not something we can just decide to do, and then do. Loving our bodies takes time. It takes patience and the willingness to open our hearts to the possibility that we are beautiful, loving beings. We may not feel beautiful. We have learned not to. The messages we have received over the years have reinforced our negative self-images repeatedly. We must begin now to give ourselves new, positive messages and to construct new images.

An exercise I often suggest to clients is to stand in front of a full-length mirror nude for five minutes. (Most of my clients strongly resist this exercise at first but when they do experiment with it they report it is very illuminating and helpful.) As you stand there, allow yourself to look at your whole body. You will most likely notice the parts of your body that you find unattractive first. You have had a lot of practice at that. But, as the time passes, please begin to notice the rest of yourself. Look at your elbows, your nose, the arches in your feet. Take in your whole self. Let yourself find at least one part of yourself to appreciate for that day. It can be an eyebrow, an ear lobe, or a wrist, for example. Each day, repeat the exercise and when you have started to see yourself a bit more fully and more tolerantly, let yourself begin to think about how your body has been treating you.

Think about the many ways this body has performed for you over the years. I am talking about *really* appreciating and getting to know your body. Become familiar with what it really looks like and appreciate how it has served you throughout your life. The process of making friends with your physical self is a worthwhile pursuit and an essential one if you are to treat yourself with respect and care. For example, if you have stretch marks that are the result of pregnancy and birth, then think of how miraculous it was to conceive and bear a child. Think of your legs and all the miles you have walked. Think about your heart and how it has been pumping blood tirelessly to all of your organs day and night for years. These are things we seldom stop to appreciate but looking at ourselves in this way can help us cultivate genuine appreciation of ourselves. *This is necessary if we are to treat ourselves in a loving way.* Our bones, our muscles, all of our body systems are part of ourselves and, although we may become ill at times, or suffer from disease or have accidents, our bodies keep serving us in the best ways they can under all circumstances.

Many of us have abused our bodies over the years. We may have starved them and then stuffed them with food. We may have given them diet pills, diuretics, and laxatives and then fed them damaging substances like caffeine, alcohol or aspartame. We may not have given them the exercise and care they have needed to perform optimally. It is not too late to begin nurturing your body and treating yourself with respect. To overcome compulsive over-eating completely, and to maintain a healthier body permanently, you must begin to cultivate a warm and friendly attitude towards your body. *It may not be perfect but it has been functioning for you since birth.* By looking at your whole self—inside and out—and appreciating yourself, you are developing the self-love necessary for the changes you plan to make.

DEALING WITH HARMFUL SUBSTANCES

Since none of us is perfect, it seems reasonable to assume that there will be times when each of us will choose to eat foods that are not good for us. It is human nature, for example, to crave sweets or caffeine at times. My experience has been that when we make a "poor" food or beverage choice, we may compound the difficulties by beating ourselves up for having "cheated" or having "been bad." This is not useful. It is vital to be able to make less than self-loving choices occasionally and then to let those choices go. If you choose to eat cake at a party, for example, and then spend several days lamenting that decision, you are setting yourself up to continue making unhealthy choices. You will continue beating yourself up and your Chew will encourage you to continue overeating to medicate your angry and disappointed feelings. It is one of the ways we punish ourselves for "being bad." This is a classic example of the Chew at work. Following is a brief discussion of some of the changes you can make that will help you to feel healthier and more in control.

It seems that eating anything sweet sets most of us up to want more sweets. I recommend omitting refined white sugar entirely from your diet. Using a bit of maple syrup, barley malt or honey is preferable if you think you must use a sweetener at all. There is also an herb called stevia that is a low calorie sweetener. This herb is estimated to be thirty times sweeter than sugar but without the calories and has been used in Paraguay for over 1500 year and in surrounding countries for centuries. You can find more information about stevia—its history, its uses, safety information, etc. by contacting Canterbury Farms which I have listed in the resource section of this book. At this time stevia has not been approved for use in the United States by the FDA.

Often women who begin working to eliminate compulsive eating with a high sugar intake learn, often to their surprise, that most foods taste as good or better with no sweetener at all. You can experiment with this. Try eating your cereal with no sugar for a few days and see if you come to appreciate the taste of the cereal itself. Once you become accustomed to leaving out the sweet taste, you may not miss it. You are likely to enjoy the taste of your food more and to notice a tremendous decrease in sugar cravings. (You also may notice you feel less depressed, jittery or anxious as well.) There may be times, however, when you do make a choice (and remember to make it a *conscious* choice) to eat sugar, perhaps at someone's birthday party or on a special holiday, for example. In that event, it is a good idea to prepare in advance for how you will handle the situation.

Understanding what is likely to occur when you eat sugar, can help you to resist the urge to follow sugar with more sugar. If you are prepared for the cravings to come, you can plan in advance how you will handle them. This process is different for each of us. For some women it is advisable to abstain totally from all sugars, for others some sugar is enjoyable and manageable. Over the years many of my clients have shared ways they have experimented with using sugar in their lives. One strategy that seems helpful to many is to plan that after you eat sugar you immediately brush your teeth to get rid of the sugary taste in your mouth and then drink plenty of cool, non-chlorinated water to flush your body systems and eliminate toxins. Sipping a cup of hot water with lemon juice and a bit of honey can help eliminate the urge to eat more sweets as well. It is also necessary to pay attention to portion size (e.g. choose a smaller piece of cake than you normally would choose) and follow the eating with some type of movement such as a short walk or a few minutes of stretching. If eating sugar feels like a set up for a binge, then plan to eat any sweets in the evening when you will soon be retiring. Although it is not advisable to eat in the evening at all (the time when we burn the fewest calories), it is better to have a small sweet then and be done with it than to have one earlier and then to continue eating sweets throughout the day.

Be aware that for many of us caffeine is also extremely addictive. If you think that you *need* coffee in the morning to wake up, if you are using coffee as a diuretic or an antidepressant or you require more and more coffee to feel your morning *high,* you are probably addicted to it to some extent. Coffee speeds up your body systems for a brief time but leaves you more tired in the long run. Think about eliminating coffee and any other chemicals that you have been putting into your system. This includes alcohol, any drugs and artificial sweeteners. If you feel that eliminating these substances all at once is too great an undertaking for you to manage at this time, choose one that you feel addicted to and start there. Cut down on that substance.

If you are addicted to drugs or alcohol, you may need professional treatment. Seek the services of an out-patient therapist or counselor who is familiar with treating addictions. If you are not able to achieve sobriety, you can enter an in-patient program to find the help you need to stop your addictive behavior. Here professionals can monitor and manage the effects of any withdrawal symptoms you experience and you can participate in therapeutic activities such as group therapy sessions and meetings. Attend Alcoholics Anonymous or Narcotics Anonymous. Many people have told me that the sober friends they made while attending these programs proved invaluable in helping them to maintain sobriety and avoid relapse. At the very least, find or form a support group for yourself. Letting go of any substance you are accustomed to using is hard and having support can determine the difference between succeeding and failing to change old, self-destructive habits.

Consider cleansing to clear chemicals out of your system. I recommend that you consult someone knowledgeable about fasting and cleansing who can supervise and support you during this experience, such as a homeopathic physician or a doctor of naturopathy. Fasting and cleansing will give you more emotional balance and great vitality but it must be done carefully. I strongly suggest that you discuss this with your medical doctor. If you are generally healthy, an occasional, brief fast can enhance your good health. If you have any medical problems, however, your physician may recommend you do not fast or that you do so only under his or her direct supervision.

If you do decide to detoxify your system, you may experience unpleasant side effects during that cleansing process, such as headaches or fatigue. These are usually positive signs that your body is ridding itself of harmful chemicals but any unusual symptoms that occur should be brought to the attention of the person supervising your cleanse. If you are interested in fasting as an option, I recommend *Juice Fasting and Detoxification* by Steve Meyerowitz. His book is comprehensive and well organized. He clearly explains fasting and methods of detoxification in depth. He tells you how to begin and what to expect and instructs you in ways to break your fast.

Included also are sections on losing weight, the psychological effects of fasting and spiritual fasting—all in all, an informative and useful guide. Each of us is different. We have different needs and desires. Each of us is unique and what "works" for one of us may not "work" for another. What we eat, how we choose to exercise our bodies (or not) and how we nurture our physical selves is up to each of us to decide. Just as what we choose to wear is a personal choice, so is the way we choose to manage *every* aspect of our lives. No one plan or one style will be appropriate for everyone.

Likewise, our nutritional needs also vary greatly. The consensus of opinion of the experts seems to be that eating a balance of nutritious foods and drinks (fresh, organic fruits and vegetables, beans and whole grains, non-chlorinated water, fresh fruit and vegetable juices and herbal teas) is our best bet. We all know on some level, that there is no nutritional value in greasy, sugary doughnuts, yet we may choose to eat these for breakfast, or not eat breakfast at all, instead of making the effort required to prepare something healthful. Either way, we sabotage ourselves. If we eat the doughnuts, we may feel sluggish, guilty and disappointed in ourselves. If we don't eat at all, we may be setting ourselves up to binge later. The idea is not to starve your body or to fill it up with foods that are calorie-dense and nutritionally poor. The idea is to experiment with your diet, making more and more self-loving decisions as time goes by.

The more you put a variety of foods that are whole, alive and nutritionally dense into your body and eliminate the processed, dead or poisoned foods, the more at peace your mind and your body will be and the less you will have cravings. Choose fresh organic fruits and vegetables and whole grains as often as possible. Eliminate processed or refined foods, white flour, white or brown sugar, and animal fats. Drink plenty of non-chlorinated water and add ample amounts of rest and exercise to your daily routine. And, most importantly, be gentle with yourself as you experiment and make gradual, lasting changes.

No one can tell you exactly what to eat, how much to eat or when to eat. Each of us is unique and my intent is to encourage you to use your intuition to make the best decisions for yourself that you can. If you begin paying close attention to how you feel when you make certain food and beverage choices, you will become more sensitive to your body and you will know what it requires to feel at its best. You will listen to your Chew less often. As you continue to experiment in this way, you will discover that the more you give your body what it *really* needs, the more at peace you will be. Your weight will stabilize at a natural, healthy place for you.

FOOD AS ADDICTION

If you have been using drugs or alcohol to cope with life situations and the accompanying feelings, you may be chemically dependent. As I mentioned in the previous section, you may need professional help to overcome your addiction. I again emphasize the importance of discussing this with a qualified drug and alcohol counselor. If you have been compulsively gambling, seeking sex partners or shopping, you would also benefit from counseling. It is hard enough to deal with compulsive eating issues without other addictions interfering. It is just about impossible to deal effectively with many addictions at the same time, especially all by yourself. With sincere desire on your part and qualified help, however, you can look at your pattern of addiction and sort it out. Then you can begin making changes that will be lasting ones.

It is common for women to identify eating concerns as a problem when they enter therapy. Frequently, however, other addictive behaviors are present as well. Often a woman will report that she begins using drugs, alcohol, compulsive shopping, etc. when she attempts to get her eating behavior under control. This makes sense especially if you are using food to dull or medicate your feelings. When you eliminate the anaesthetic of food, your feelings are likely to surface. If food is not available as a way to deny or avoid these new feelings, you may search for some other way to turn them off. To be successful at *Taming your Chew* you will have to look at your personal complex of addictions and plan strategies to eliminate them.

I had a client who was struggling valiantly with her compulsive eating problems. She would turn to alcohol, however, whenever she stopped binge-eating behavior for any period of time. She and her husband would argue constantly about her drinking. The marital relationship would suffer and eventually she would return to food for consolation. This was a self-defeating cycle for her and for her husband as well. Only after they had talked about their relationship in counseling and taken steps to improve it was the woman able to concentrate on stopping her compulsive behavior.

You may be using food to mask other issues and to dull uncomfortable feelings in your life. Counseling can help you focus on these feelings and to experience them, understand them and learn healthier ways to cope with them. If we medicate with any substance to avoid what we are feeling—as we may have learned to do early on—we remain out of touch with ourselves and our real needs. If we attempt to ignore the feelings we have, we will eat to suppress them again and again. Our feelings surface to help us. They are important messengers who bring us valuable information about our lives and ourselves. It is *crucial* that we learn to listen to and appreciate them. We will visit this topic again in the section on *Healing the Emotional Self.*

Thousands of women have found help with addictions within twelve step programs such as Alcoholics Anonymous, Narcotics Anonymous, Overeaters Anonymous or Adult Children of Alcoholics. There are supportive programs like these for people with most addictions (e.g. gambling, sex, spending). Within these groups women have their feelings and experiences validated. They find out that they are not alone and discover that millions of others suffer with the same difficulties and feelings. These groups also supply the education and support necessary to overcome addiction. When we suffer alone with our feelings and problems, they quickly become unmanageable. When we open ourselves to receive help and care from others and realize that we don't have to struggle alone, difficulties shift into perspective. If you try to isolate and correct self-destructive eating patterns by yourself, you are setting yourself up to fail. If you do not accept support from some source, you will easily become discouraged and frustrated and food will continue to serve as your consolation.

With support, things will not seem quite so overwhelming and you will be able to focus on making healthy, self-loving choices in all areas of your life. If you use your support system, think in terms of your "whole" self and take your whole lifestyle into account, you will be able to initiate the changes necessary for healthy growth. If you try to change addictive behaviors without considering your environmental, intellectual, spiritual and emotional needs you cannot be successful. Changing one part of the whole effects all of the parts. If you try to eat differently but continue other self-abusive practices, it won't be long before your Chew will take over. Think in terms of getting healthier in the bigger picture. Consider any addictive behaviors you struggle with and plan ways to work on eliminating them. *Think of this time as an opportunity to make changes in many areas of your life. First consider what your physical, emotional, societal and spiritual needs are and then make changes accordingly.*

EXPLORING NONTRADITIONAL WAYS OF HEALING

Today there are many beneficial alternative services that can help you to heal physically as well as emotionally and spiritually. Following is a list of some of the services currently available to help you on your journey towards optimum health. I urge you to read through this list and to familiarize yourself with it. You might also consult *The American Holistic Health Association Complete Guide to Alternative Medicine* by William Collinge, M.P.H., Ph.D. Then, armed with knowledge about specific types of alternative health care available, you can experiment with different types of service. Think of this as an opportunity and an adventure. Notice what sparks your interest and trust your intuitive voice to direct you to the types of work that will be most helpful for you. Healing and nurturing your body, mind and spirit is primary if you are to stop eating compulsively and there are many people working in exciting and innovative ways who can help you to accomplish this.

One word of caution: there are many ethical and reputable holistic practitioners who are competing for your service. There are also others who may not have your best interests in mind. Use your discretion when you choose to sample any type of care (medical, psychological, spiritual, etc.). Ask for references. Ask where, when and how this practitioner was trained and what experience they have had in the field. Make a list of questions you want to ask and then interview him or her over the telephone prior to scheduling a meeting. If, over the telephone (or later, in person) you feel uneasy in any way, do not schedule (or, if you are already there, terminate the session and leave). *You* are the consumer. *You* are the one in control and *you* know best.

If you try a service and do not find it to be helpful, try another. Not every service is helpful for every person. Also, a service that does not "fit" for you at this particular time in your life may prove to be exactly what you need at a different time. Life is a learning process after all. Remember, there are no mistakes, only lessons.

Mind/Body Interventions

Art Therapy—offers a synthesis of psychotherapy and art. Clients use the medium of art materials as a vehicle for self-expression and exploration which can lead to greater expression of feeling, self-understanding, acceptance and health.

Biofeedback—uses various instruments to give information about bodily processes such as blood pressure and heart rate—clients learn ways to use breathing techniques to lower these body systems for enhanced relaxation, stress reduction, management of chronic pain and other disorders.

Dance Therapy—uses movement to help clients access and express feelings, leading to increased awareness of themselves on all levels—emotionally, physically, and spiritually.

Guided Imagery—combines deep breathing and relaxation while using the mind's ability to imagine sights, sounds, smells or movements to induce specific reactions in the body or to encourage changes in a client's emotional outlook.

Humor—evokes healing energies through the use of humor and play—helps people to relax and maintain perspective in their lives.

Hypnotherapy—employs deep breathing with hypnotic suggestions to enable clients to access inner resources—useful at times for controlling pain, eliminating self-destructive habits or recovering suppressed memories.

Meditation—uses breathing and repetition of a sound, word, phrase, prayer or muscular activity to minimize distracting thoughts, and passive return to the repetition when distracting thoughts do occur. This practice often helps clients become more in touch with their spirituality.

Music Therapy—uses music and its influence to aid in physiological, psychological and emotional integration of the individual during treatment of an illness or disability. Uses music to effect changes in behaviors, emotions or physiology.

Prayer Therapy—incorporates prayer by individuals and groups to ask for help with healing on physical, emotional and spiritual levels.

Psychotherapy—takes various forms depending upon orientation of the therapist. Interview prospective therapists and question them about their philosophy and methods of treatment.

Relaxation—trains one to relax the body and quiet the mind through the use of deep breathing and awareness focusing techniques.

Support Groups—helps with the healing process by teaching members they are not alone and providing opportunities for members to talk about their experiences and feelings. People can heal through these connections with others and thus become more connected to their own experience and feelings.

Yoga—integrates body, mind and spirit utilizing movement and breath and may include instructions in lifestyle changes to facilitate healing and enhance health.

Qigong—(chee-goong) emphasizes breathing, meditation and both stationery and moving postures to enhance the flow of Chi (chee) energy throughout the body.

Tai Chi—(a style of Qigong) uses meditation and slow movement to affect flow of Chi and bring about physical self-awareness.

Alternative Systems of Medical Practice

Acupuncture—uses insertion of special needles into acupuncture points along the fourteen meridians of the body to correct and rebalance flow of energy throughout the body.

Ayurveda—draws from medicinal practice of India and is over 6000 years old—views individuals according to their particular constitution and includes specific recommendations for diet, exercise, herbal treatments, massage and cleansing techniques to heal body, mind and spirit.

Homeopathy—uses "law of similars" or "like cures like" to make remedies that are effective in treating various physical and emotional conditions.

Naturopathy—follows premise of "do no harm"—avoids drugs and/or surgery whenever possible. Utilizes a number of alternative therapies.

Traditional Chinese medicine—holds the philosophy that the medicine is preventive in nature and views the body as a reflection of the natural world. Wellness is a function of a balanced, harmonious flow of Chi energy through the body and illness or disease is the result of disturbances in this flow of energy. Methods used include meditation, acupuncture, visualization, relaxation, breathing exercises, postures, massage and manipulation, fasting, dietary recommendations, and herbal treatments.

Other Healing Practices

Acupressure—uses applied pressure along meridians to alter energy flow, remove energy blockages and strengthen Chi energy.

Shiatsu—(Japanese technique) similar to acupressure to encourage flow of energy.

Alexander Technique—uses body work to correct posture and movement patterns and to release painful muscle tension.

Aston-Patterning—tailors the Alexander Technique to particular characteristics of a client's body.

Chiropractic Medicine—operates using a holistic approach to health. Believes in the body's inherent ability to heal itself by reestablishing an unobstructed flow of nerve impulses between the brain and the rest of the body. Practitioners believe the body seeks homeostasis (balance) and cannot achieve this when the body is out of alignment. "Straight" chiropractors use manipulation of the spine to free nerve channels and facilitate the movement of energy. "Mixers" do the same but also use manipulation of muscle systems and various other alternative procedures (e.g. electrical stimulation, ice, heat, ultrasound, traction). Mixers also may use various forms of massage, trigger point manipulation, craniopathy, sacro-occipital technique, applied kinesiology, exercise, vitamin and mineral supplementation, nutrition and dietary alterations. Used for neuromuscular conditions and may also be useful for many other ailments.

Feldenkrais Method—uses verbal instructions, touch and movement to teach new patterns to improve posture, movement and breathing.

Massage Therapy—manipulates soft tissues of body to reduce tension and stress, improve circulation, aid healing of muscle and soft tissue, control pain and promote overall well-being. There are a wide range of massage techniques. Call to interview practitioners and ask about the style of massage they offer.

Osteopathy—corrects musculoskeletal problems to improve overall body function. Also considers psychological factors, lifestyle, and diet.

Reflexology—manipulates areas of the feet and hands that correspond with a particular organ or zone in the upper body to stimulate internal organs and to bring body into balance. Used to relieve stress, headaches, sinus problems, constipation, insomnia, hypertension, anxiety, and premenstrual syndrome.

Reiki—Uses the "laying on of hands" to direct life force energy into the body. Used for stress reduction, overall well-being and to promote healing.

Rolfing—(structural integration) aligns the body in ways necessary for physical and emotional health. Uses combination of massage and movement.

Hellerwork—(off shoot of Rolfing) combines touch and movement to teach stress-free ways to perform activities.

Therapeutic Touch—does not use physical contact—hands are placed 2" to 6" from client and moved in graceful, sweeping motions over the body to detect blockages in the energy field. Healer focuses energy to client to replenish, balance and unblock energy flow.

Trager Psychophysical Integration—utilizes gentle touch, rhythmic rocking, shaking and exercises to identify and correct tension patterns that affect posture and movement (particularly good for neuromuscular problems from injuries, Multiple Sclerosis or Muscular Dystrophy).

Myotherapy—uses deep massage to reduce tension and pain.

Polarity—uses subtle touch or holding on to specific pressure points and joints, massage, breathing, hydrotherapy, exercise and reflexology.

Aromatherapy—uses essential oils extracted from plants to promote relaxation and relieve certain symptoms—used in diffusers, baths, massage oils, compresses.

Hydrotherapy—utilizes wraps, sprays, douches, steam room, sauna, hot or cold baths, whirlpools, sitz baths to stimulate immune system and detoxify the body.

Orthomolecular Medicine—uses vitamins, minerals and amino acids to treat specific conditions (asthma, heart disease, depression, schizophrenia—also for general good health).

Herbal Medicine

Today many people are using herbs and herbal preparations in lieu of traditional medications to treat various physical and emotional complaints.

Herbal Therapy—uses herbs made from plants to treat mild or chronic ailments—some herbs can be toxic, so please seek guidance before using herbs.

Chinese Herbal Therapy—recommends various Chinese herbal combinations to correct energy imbalances and to treat specific ailments. (Again, please seek guidance from an experienced herbalist.)

A complete guide to herbal medicine is far beyond the scope of this book, but some books that you may find useful if you would like to use herbs to treat physical or emotional ailments are:

Natural Health, Natural Medicine—Andrew Weil, M.D.
The Natural Remedy Book for Women—Diane Stein
Prescription for Nutritional Healing—James F. Balch, M.D. &
    Phyllis A. Balch, C.N.C.
Healthy Healing—Linda Rector Page, N.D.,Ph.D.
Holistic Herbal—David Hoffmann
*The American Holistic Association Complete Guide to
    Alternative Medicine*—William Collinge, M.P.H.,Ph.D.

Also useful for many people are Bach Flower Remedies. These
are not used directly for physical illness, but instead attend to psychic
symptoms. These remedies work to strengthen the life force and
remove energy blockages when the client is experiencing certain dis-
comforts. There are 38 different remedies that can be purchased at
most health stores. In Diane Stein's book, *The Natural Remedy Book
for Women* you can find a thorough explanation of flower essences
and an extensive list of remedies that are helpful for different conditions.

Diet, nutrition and lifestyle changes are often indicated to help
people come into emotional, physical and spiritual balance. There are
many ways to work on this. You can explore different nutrition plans,
such as macrobiotics or various vegetarian diets, and consult with a
professional to determine vitamin and mineral supplements that will
help you. You may explore juicing as one avenue towards increased
good health and vitality and/or find out about various cleansing practices.

As you consider any form of self-help, follow your intuitive voice.
You cannot do everything and so you must carefully choose directions
you would like to explore further. Experiment. Think of this as a
journey towards greater health, balance and serenity. Life is ever-
changing, ever-unfolding, ever-challenging. There is no way to do
any of this perfectly. So, please release those persistent, self-expectations of perfection. They are impossible to achieve and serve only to
keep you endlessly frustrated and plagued with fears of inadequacy.
You are not inadequate. You are human. So, relax, experiment, and
open yourself to trying new things. Your Chew will become more
peaceful and calm as you become more peaceful and calm.

Reflections

Chapter VIII

Healing the Emotional Self

LOVING OUR LITTLE GIRL

SOMEWHERE along the line each of us has been hurt in some way. Being alive means having a wide range of experiences and some of these are more or less pleasant than others. Some help us feel proud of ourselves and build self-esteem, others do the opposite. We all enter this world as sparkling little souls. To know this you only have to look into the eyes of any tiny child. They are filled with excitement and wonder, as were our eyes at one time. What happens then as we grow that causes so many of us to lose that sparkle and sense of joy? Where do our feelings of wonder, magic and adventure go? Where does our tiny child go? What happened to her? Does she still exist? Can she come back?

When a little girl is violated in some way, she begins to hide her true self. As protection, she must conceal her feelings from those who might blame her and harm her further. She pushes her strongest emotions safely and deeply inside. She *must* do this to survive in a confusing and hurtful world. That little girl who came into the world bursting with good feelings and trust learns quickly that the world is not always a safe place. Perhaps she begins to wonder what *she* has done to cause others to treat her so poorly. "Surely if I am a good girl, people will love me and treat me well. If people treat me in a 'bad' way, then *I* must be bad." Children are very concrete and they see themselves as the center of the universe. They imagine that they are the cause of everything. All of us had to pass through this vulnerable time to get to adulthood and all of us had our basic sense of self-worth shaped by experiences along the way.

Many of us have been abused. Some of us have experienced severe physical, sexual and emotional violations. Some of us have had our spirits trampled. Through these experiences as children we became convinced that we were "bad" in some way. Then we carried those feelings and beliefs—that "old baggage"—with us from times past into the present. The feeling that something was wrong with us as children was our reality then. We were too little to understand that we had done nothing wrong. The adults in our life were responsible for our pain but we felt 'bad.' We could not blame those who were caring for us. That would have been far too scary. After all, they had power over our very survival. They were our caretakers and protectors and yet they were hurting or neglecting us. There was no other way to make sense of this other than to take in the message that we were the "bad" ones. It had to be us. It surely could not have been *them*.

Many of us carry that old reality subconsciously into present time. We may still walk around thinking and feeling deep within our core self that we are "bad." We may still think on some level that we caused our own abuse and therefore we need to continue to punish ourselves for it. It may still be too frightening to name our childhood abusers and to put our anger outside of ourselves and onto them where it belongs. The same result most likely occurred if our perpetrator was not a relative. We may have been abused by a babysitter, a neighbor, a friend of the family or an older child in our neighborhood, for example. No matter who violated us or when it happened, we may have filled with shame and self-hatred then and the feelings of shame and guilt persist today. We keep punishing ourselves for being "bad" and we often do so with our food abusive behavior.

If we have lived as survivors of rape or battering, for example, we may carry our guilt and pain around with us every day. The "habit" of blaming ourselves for *anything* that is bad or goes wrong seems, in my experience, to come naturally to many women. We are ready to take on the burdens of others and to sacrifice our self-esteem for their good. Heaven forbid that when someone is hurtful to us we tell them we are angry and to stop hurting us! We might hurt their feelings! Better that we hold in our feelings, continue to see ourselves as responsible for their behavior, make sure they are OK and then go eat a dozen cupcakes. Sound familiar? Make sense? Have you ever noticed how often you turn to food after denying your own experience and feelings and expending all your energy on others?

Abuse can mean many things. It may be blatant harm done to us or it may consist of subtle messages we received about who we are and what we do. *Any disrespectful act or remark that is damaging to us is abusive.* Some women I have worked with have suffered much abuse and never considered their experience as hurtful to them until we began to explore their experiences and pull out those that set them up for self-abusive messages and behaviors as adults. If you think that some of your compulsive eating behavior is wrapped up in negative feelings about yourself, please talk about this with a counselor, minister, therapist or some person who can help you to sort it out and to stop blaming yourself for your abusive experiences. If you try to love yourself and nurture yourself while secretly harboring feelings of self-hatred, guilt, shame and fear, your efforts will be futile. You were not responsible for things other people said and did to you. You *must* free yourself from feeling "bad" or responsible.

Besides talking to an appropriate person, please take any opportunity to nurture the child within yourself. Buy yourself a stuffed animal. It doesn't matter if you are nine or ninety, a furry little animal to cuddle and talk to can help when you are alone, scared or sad (and we *all* have those feelings at times). Stuffed animals (and some pets) make great listeners, love to be hugged, never invalidate or argue with you and bring back a bit of the magic that you may have lost as a child. Choose one carefully. It should be soft and tug a bit at your heart.

Let yourself play. Use your creative, expressive self. Get some finger paints or crayons and big sheets of paper and scribble, write or draw. Smear glue on your artwork and sprinkle glitter on it. Grab some Play-Doh or clay and pound it, roll it, shape it, toss it, or do anything else that strikes your fancy. Walk barefoot upon the earth. Run through a sprinkler. Be daring. Dance. Giggle. Do something different. Play for the sake of playing. Enjoy being!

When I lead workshops on women's psychology or compulsive eating issues, I ask the women who attend what they do to *play*. Usually they look at me and at each other as if I have spoken in Swahili or Greek. They will generally fidget a bit and finally someone will meekly offer an answer such as, "I read." Well, reading can be relaxing and fun but it also can be an escape from living your life.

When I speak of "play," I am talking about something quite the opposite. I am speaking about doing things to feel alive and to encourage your child-like feelings to surface. Go to a playground and hop on a swing. Skip through a meadow or along a beach. Roll in a pile of autumn leaves. Make a mud pie. Chew bubble gum and blow the biggest bubbles you can. Pop it on the tip of your nose. Take off your shoes and feel the air between your toes. Be courageous. Make a mess. Stamp your feet. Allow yourself to be a little bit less rigid and have a little (or a lot) more fun. Read *Succulent Wild Woman: Dancing with your Wonder-full Self,* by Sark. Let her take you on a riotous adventure. Her book is all about playing and being outrageous and daring and free. It is about lightness and spirit. I highly recommend it!

Read some of the books written on caring for and healing your inner child but don't get so hung up on this that you get stuck in the past. Visit your past, but don't stay there. It is important to heal and part of the healing process is learning how to take care of yourself in present time. Acknowledge your hurts, express your anger about them and then move lovingly on. Don't waste too much of your precious time on people and events from your past. This process is different for each of us and, as I said earlier, it is most helpful to have someone who is qualified and objective to help you through the process. There is no one correct way to work on these old issues; each of us is different and each of us needs to honor our own experiences and feelings and work through them at a comfortable pace and in our own unique ways. Carolyn Myss, in her audiotape *Why People Don't Heal,* depicts therapy as a boat which you get into to negotiate your way through a troubled time—to cross turbulent waters, for example. She points out that sometimes people stay in the boat and fail to move on in present time. So, please seek help if you have old issues impeding your progress but please don't forget to get out of the boat when the necessary ride is over.

The important thing to be aware of is that the negative feelings we have about ourselves are natural given the life experiences we have had and to realize that one result of these feelings is anxiety. Anxiety is uncomfortable and we have learned well to suppress uncomfortable feelings with food. Our Chew knows this and wants us to continue doing so. We don't have to listen, however. We can choose something different.

Rethinking old beliefs and nurturing our little girl inside can free us from the pain and guilt we have carried for a lifetime. Let yourself begin today to be more loving, tender and gentle with yourself. No matter what you have thought in the past, allow yourself to entertain the possibility that you are special and lovable. Even if you don't feel that way at first, look into the mirror and tell yourself that it is so. *As you shed old negative beliefs about yourself, you will rediscover the sparkling, curious, precious little being that you have always been. Then you will be truly ready to nurture your body and your spirit.*

CELEBRATING OUR SEXUALITY

Sexuality is a sensitive area for most of us to discuss. It is hard to talk about, write about or think about and uncomfortable for most of us to address. Sexuality means different things to each of us and there are as many ways to think about it as there are women in the world. We are all sexual beings. We were born with sexual feelings and instincts but most of us were never taught that these feelings are natural and beautiful. Many of us learned instead that our bodies and our urges for sexual expression and gratification were "dirty" or "bad" in some way.

Today as I watch my grown children parent their children, I am both delighted and impressed to see issues about my grandchildren's bodies and sexual feelings handled quite differently. One day when my daughter was visiting with her son (then two years old) he began to touch his "private" area. My daughter lovingly told him that it was fine to touch himself but that he should only do this in a private place. She told him he could go into the bathroom or his bedroom to do so. She was open to answering any questions he had and made sure that he understood both sides of the issue.

Each of my grandchildren has learned about privacy and the right to enjoy their bodies in this natural way. They are able to express their feelings and not hide them away in shame. They have also learned when touching themselves is, and is not, appropriate and acceptable and they have begun to develop clear boundaries. Sexual concerns have been handled nonjudgementally. Their parents did not act horrified or scold them for having natural urges and feelings. There was no shame attached to their bodies or to their pleasurable sexual feelings and expression. These children are growing up knowing that it is acceptable to enjoy their bodies and to be fully alive. All of them are able to talk about their body parts and to freely ask questions of the adults they trust. This is as it should be. Most of us, however, did not receive the same encouragement to feel good about our bodies and about sexual feelings. Most of us received exactly the opposite: messages that directly fostered shame and guilt.

One client shared a particularly painful example of her introduction to sexual shame and guilt. As a small child, she learned that her natural urges to enjoy sexual feelings were unacceptable. She learned this through the direct experiencing of her mother's fear of sexuality. Through the following experience it became clear to her that there was no place for her sexual feelings to fit comfortably into her life. This client recalled being very small, perhaps only three or four and spending the night at her grandparent's house. She was excited to be sleeping there and was to sleep in a twin bed with her mother. She recalled feeling safe and relaxed as she curled closely next to her mother's warmth. She began instinctively to touch her genitals as she drifted off to sleep. Suddenly her mother startled her by demanding in a loud voice, "What are you doing?" Even at such a tender age it was clearly communicated through her mother's tone that she was doing something quite unacceptable. By talking about this experience, she was able to see that seeds of shame and guilt had been deeply planted at that moment.

The messages many of us received as children about ourselves as sexual beings were most likely negative and confusing and they set the tone for our attitudes and beliefs later as adults. We were not urged to celebrate our sexual or passionate feelings. No one encouraged us to embrace that creative, vibrant part of ourselves. Instead, we were punished and judged. Sometimes we were directly told *not* to be sexual beings. At other times the messages were subtle—delivered by a word, a gesture or a glance. The end result was the same: confusion, shame and guilt.

Most of us were never told to "do it somewhere else." Instead we were told not to do it at all. Since sexual feelings are natural, we had them. Being told not to have feelings that we cannot help but have is confusing and destructive. It is unlikely that anyone could grow up respecting and appreciating his or her sexuality under these circumstances. Additionally, the messages are quite different for each gender. When many of us were growing up—and it may not be much different today—there was a blatant double standard. Boys were often congratulated for sexual performance. Having sexual experiences made them "men." For girls, however, the same experiences earned the label of "slut" or "whore." A girl was told that if a boy became aroused it was her fault. Girls were encouraged to act in sexual, provocative ways by messages they received from society, the media, etc. But, at the same time, they were told to save their virginity for their marital partner. Girls were given all the responsibility and all of the shame. You may have heard the expression that "men want their women to be virgins in the living room but whores in the bedroom." Just how does one *do* that? Talk about mixed, confusing messages!

We have considered how our feelings about our bodies and ourselves are intricately woven into our patterns of eating. If your feelings about yourself as a sexual being are confusing and shame-based, please locate someone you can be comfortable talking about these feelings with, such as a counselor or a good friend. You are most likely carrying around old baggage. If you feel anxious thinking and talking about your body or about sexual concerns you are most likely harboring unnecessary fear, guilt and shame. Educate yourself. There are many books that can help you to explore and further understand your sexuality. One book, *For Yourself: The Fulfillment of Female Sexuality* by Lonnie Barbach has proven useful to a number of my clients.

Find support! Talk with a few people you trust and feel close to about your sexual attitudes, feelings and experiences. Most likely they will be able to understand. Knowing that you are not alone and that others share your concerns and feelings helps. By talking about your sexuality, you demystify it and decrease any feelings of guilt, anxiety, fear or shame that you have been harboring. This is a big step towards emotional, physical and spiritual health and will help you to eliminate compulsive eating behavior. So, do all you can to take control over this aspect of your life. *Being a sexual being is natural. It is a beautiful, spiritual part of each of us and is to be celebrated—not hidden away under a blanket of anxiety, guilt and shame.*

SETTING BOUNDARIES

For years I heard people talk about setting clear boundaries and I had no idea what they were talking about. This was not something we ever discussed in my family of origin. The whole concept was foreign to me and any readings I found directly dealing with this topic were unclear and did little to help me figure it out. I asked professors and peers to explain boundaries but no one told me anything concrete to really clarify the term. So, I observed people who seemed healthy and well adjusted and I listened carefully to them. I watched other people make themselves and their needs top priority and gradually I began to get some idea of what people meant by "clear, firm boundaries."

Having boundaries means many different things. It means feeling good about ourselves and setting clear limits with others. It means saying what we really mean and then sticking to it. It means not allowing ourselves to be taken advantage of and expressing our true feelings. It means taking responsibility for ourselves and our feelings and not for everyone else and their feelings. In short, it means being true to ourselves. Sounds simple, does it not? But, no, it is very hard. It appears particularly difficult for women because we have been taught so well to consider others and their needs above ourselves and our own needs.

This is an important topic for each of us to consider. If we do not understand what " healthy boundaries" are we will not be able create them and maintain them. If we don't create and maintain them, we will feel confused, unhappy and anxious and, we are likely to search for food to anesthetize ourselves and soothe our discomfort. Having clear, healthy boundaries is essential to feeling in control of our lives and to eliminating compulsive eating behavior permanently.

Take a few minutes to think about exactly what some of your limits and boundaries are and how you can enforce them to protect and care for yourself. Close your eyes and take a few deep, full breaths. Think about the ways you give your energy to other people and things throughout the day. When do you reserve time and energy for yourself? Imagine yourself going through a typical day considering your own desires, feelings and needs before jumping to meet the demands put upon you by others. Can you imagine yourself setting limits and communicating your feelings clearly and assertively to others in your life? At first you may feel selfish focusing your attention on yourself, but please stay with the exercise and see if you can discover at least one area of your life where you can make even a small change. Start there—for example, by telling your neighbor that you are no longer willing to watch her child every afternoon for no compensation. Experiment with saying "no" in a clear voice. If you do this, you will be surprised at how empowered you will feel as bit by bit you assume more control of your time and your energy.

Having healthy boundaries means many other things as well. It means trusting appropriately. It means entering into and building any relationship step by step. Sometimes we may think in black and white terms, either not trusting at all or trusting completely before we really get to know the other person. Have you ever shared intimate details of your life with someone you just met? Have you fallen in love at first sight? Have you felt overwhelmed by another or totally preoccupied with another? These are all signs of unclear, unhealthy, "fuzzy" boundaries. When we have clear boundaries, we go slowly and move into any relationship paying careful attention to our inner voices. We don't distrust or fully trust immediately. We become intimate one step at a time, all the while asking ourselves if this is a healthy connection for us to put our energy into. We stay focused on our own growth and needs and we make self-loving choices about relationships (as we do about food).

Having clear boundaries means respecting ourselves. We weigh the consequences of our actions and maintain our personal values whether others agree with them or not. We become sexually involved only when we feel comfortable doing so. When we do choose to be sexual, we concentrate largely on our own pleasure rather than performing primarily to please or take care of our partner and we say "no" to any advance, touch, sex, gift, food, etc. that we don't want. Likewise, we respect others. We ask another before touching them and we do not take advantage of, or exploit others, in any way. We clearly communicate our wants and our needs and we treat ourselves and others fairly and lovingly.

Being clear means talking to ourselves and others gently, honestly, assertively, respectfully and lovingly. It means staying centered on ourselves and nurturing a positive attitude. It means using our sense of humor and being our own loving, nurturing parent. If we fail to do these things, life is murky and difficult much of the time. Our needs get mixed up with other people's needs and we end up giving up parts of ourselves to take care of others. We may set aside our plans or goals because we view others' needs as more important and we focus our energy on helping them to reach their goals. We become resentful and then we suppress our anger and become anxious. Our Chew goes wild. We feel ravenous and then overeat to calm our nerves.

This is what we were taught as children. Many, if not most of us, grew up in families where clear boundaries were never modeled or taught to us. Most likely our parents were never taught about boundaries and their importance. They couldn't explain or model clear boundaries for us if they didn't know what they were. We were left on our own to figure it out for ourselves. As I found this topic confusing, most of my clients initially do as well. A central part of anyone's treatment for compulsive eating behavior is learning what boundaries are and how to set and maintain them. For many this is difficult and specific instruction is needed on how to communicate, how to be assertive (not aggressive) and how to say "no."

Because women are socialized to be passive, to please others, and to put personal needs aside, being assertive and clear does not come easily. It is often extremely difficult. Some have trouble at first just saying the word "no." If you find that this is an area you struggle with in your life, I recommend that you enroll in an assertiveness training group or a therapy group that focuses on helping members to learn how to set and maintain clear boundaries. You can call therapists in your area, hospitals, mental health centers or colleges that cater to adult students. Find out what's available in your area and take advantage of it. If you can't locate the type of service you need, go to a library or bookstore and locate self-help books on assertiveness. Perhaps you and other women friends could read these books at the same time and get together to talk about them. You might arrange meetings to discuss your readings and to support each other while making the necessary changes in your attitudes and behaviors. *Even though it may seem awkward or scary at first, it is crucial to be true to yourself and to set boundaries that feel appropriate and safe for you. If you do not, you will continue to eat your way through the confusing and painful feelings you will experience.*

COMMUNICATING ASSERTIVELY

Communicating our thoughts and feelings honestly and directly is difficult for most of us. We have been taught to tailor our words and our behaviors to please others and to meet their needs, often at the exclusion of our own. I find that women who come to me with eating issues invariably have difficulty expressing themselves verbally in many situations. Because relationships are of paramount importance to us and because we fear that others may become angry or even abandon us, we may sometimes sit in silence, holding in our true feelings. If we are to feel good about ourselves, we need to express ourselves even when our opinion may be at odds with another's. Perhaps you can think of a situation where you held feelings inside. Maybe you were angry about something but decided to "let it go" because "it wasn't worth making a fuss." Did you later turn to potato chips or chocolate? Did your Chew become agitated? Just begin to notice.

Carry a small notepad with you for a few weeks. When you feel the urge to eat, take a minute to open your notepad. Close your eyes, take a deep breath, and ask yourself, "what am I feeling right now?" Write your feelings down and then ask yourself, "how will eating help me to cope with this feeling?" Over time, you will see that food is simply the vehicle you have been using to deny or repress your feelings. If you learn to deal directly with the feelings instead, you will no longer be tempted to turn to food to medicate them.

Recently a client, who was ending her therapy, told me that of all the work we had done, the most helpful piece for her was making the connection between her feelings and her urge to eat. Carrying her notepad and writing before she ate helped her to recognize the ways she was using food to cope with various difficult feelings. Armed with this knowledge, she empowered herself to make healthier, more self-loving choices. In this way, she set firm, clear boundaries, built self-confidence, boosted her self-esteem, and thus stopped thoughtless, compulsive eating behaviors. She was finally able to lose the weight she had been struggling with since childhood. (She *Tamed her Chew.*)

Communicating effectively and being assertive are essential behaviors and they are seldom taught to us. Many of us did not have parents who modeled assertive, clear behavior; nor were we encouraged to go outside of our homes to acquire these skills. Think about all the messages we receive to nurture others and to be compliant, even passive. Where on earth would we learn to be assertive? We may know some women who have risen into positions of power in our society. These women, who might serve as role models for us, are often unappreciated and viewed by others in our culture as "pushy," aggressive, or abrasive. We may want to achieve our goals and speak our minds, but the fear of being seen in this way stops us. We don't want to be considered "pushy" or aggressive do we? We don't want to risk disapproval.

Often when we begin to experiment with expressing ourselves honestly, we fear we are being inappropriate. We may think we are coming across as aggressive, and we can sound a bit aggressive at first. If we have been passive and compliant most of our lives, we may sound aggressive when we first try to assert ourselves. This is because when anyone begins to practice any new behavior, they are naturally awkward and tense and may go a bit too far in first attempts to assert themselves. We may speak a bit too loudly or harshly because we feel nervous. With practice, however, we become more proficient and the behaviors feel more natural. We learn to choose our words and to modulate our tone and volume of voice appropriately. Expressing ourselves is like that—harder at first, easier as we become accustomed to it. I highly recommend a complete course in assertiveness or communication skills and will make a few basic suggestions to get you started.

My first recommendation is that you educate yourself. There are many self-help books on the market that focus on communication skills and the art of being assertive. Reading about the experiences of others and about ways to begin practicing new skills can help you find the courage necessary to experiment with new, healthier behaviors in your own life situation. Community colleges or adult education organizations offer classes, courses, workshops or lectures to help you learn basic assertiveness or communications skills. Libraries may lend books or audiotapes and videotapes on these topics. Find out what resources are available in your area and take full advantage of them.

Some of us grew up with a few positive female role models in our world, others of us had absolutely none. If you have particular difficulty saying "no" to others, setting clear, firm boundaries or putting your own needs before others' needs, please consider finding a therapist in your area who can help you to develop healthier ways to interact with the people in your life. Many of us received an abundance of negative messages when we were little girls. Perhaps we were sexually, emotionally or physically abused and our self-esteem was trampled as a result. Maybe we were sensitive to being unappreciated or devalued by others. At the very least we were all bombarded with negative images and messages from our culture. It is very difficult to grow up surrounded by this negativity and emerge as confident, articulate, assertive women. Making changes is always challenging. A supportive, nonjudgmental therapist can help you to look at why assertive behavior is difficult for you and help you to move past these blockages to a more secure and confident way of being.

Additionally, it is necessary to feel the support of others when you make life changes and I cannot emphasize strongly enough the importance of having a support group. For many of us, family members can help us enormously with their encouragement and care. For others, primary support may need to come from outside of our home and family. Peers, especially if they are going through some of the same struggles as we are, can be invaluable. Optimally, you will find ample support within your family system as well as outside with your peers. If that is not the case, at the very least please line up one or two friends to check in with regularly (at least two or three times a week). If you can find a therapy or support group in your area, consider joining. If not, consider starting a support network of your own. *You will need to talk about your fears, your feelings and your progress with someone. Trying to do it all by yourself is a set-up for failure and an opportunity for your Chew to rule.*

SEEING WITH HUMOR

One resource many of us do not take advantage of often enough is our sense of humor. Laughter is a release of emotion and tension and helps us to cope with our stressful schedules and lives. According to Loretta LaRoche, well-known comedian, teacher and founder of Wellness Associates, Plymouth, Massachusetts, there are many benefits from using our sense of humor. When we laugh we increase our heart rate, raise our blood pressure and accelerate our breathing. This leads to greater oxygen consumption, increased energy and relaxation. We give our stomach and facial muscles a workout and we relax the muscles we are not using at the time. People who appreciate and enjoy the humor in their lives are generally more relaxed, more creative, more flexible and better able to cope with problems. They live longer lives, have less illness and lower stress levels.

We live in a high-tech, fast-paced, high-tension world and we become like pressure cookers holding in emotion. If we do not release our feelings somehow, we build tension in our bodies and then race to the refrigerator for relief. You may notice that when you are feeling out of control around food it is because you are tense in some way. It is not when you feel relaxed and happy that you pounce on your food and cram it forcefully into your mouth. It is when you are looking for something to "take the edge off," to help you cope with certain feelings or situations. Incorporating more opportunities for laughter and fun into your life can help you to develop a more positive attitude about life in general. This will help you to stay in control of your behavior more often and to cope more effectively with difficulties as they arise.

Sometimes we take life too seriously. Even a minor annoyance can assume huge proportions. It is helpful at times to back up, take a deep breath and ask yourself, "How important is this?" We may spend our day fretting and fuming over our negative circumstances and we totally miss the joy and beauty available in the present. You are the only one who suffers when you put your precious energy into harboring negative feelings about someone else. The other person is probably having a fine day and spending very little time concerned about how you are doing or feeling. If you allow negative thoughts about someone to ruin your day, you are giving that person your power. You give up the right to enjoy yourself and your life and you find yourself stewing about things in the past that you have absolutely no control over.

A client of mine was divorced some time ago. For a long time, she focused much of her attention on how badly her ex-husband had betrayed her and hurt her. She reflected on the past and obsessed about the pain that he had caused her and she was unable to focus her energy on enjoying any aspects of her life in the present. She is just now beginning to understand that he has gone on with his life. He is moving forward, working, being productive and he is oblivious to the pain she has wrapped herself in. She is starting to pull her attention into the present more often. By reminding herself to stay in present time, taking life a bit less seriously and giving herself positive messages she is letting go of the negative, destructive thoughts with which she has been torturing herself for months. As she lets go of thoughts of him and focuses on her own well-being, she feels happier and more energized. She is laughing more and appreciating the humor in her own life. She is reclaiming her personal power and she is able to relax and enjoy herself.

We all have the ability to change our attitudes and to focus our attention in either positive or negative directions. *It really is up to us.* We may sometimes feel victimized and hopeless, that is inevitable, but we do have choices about how we respond in any situation. Even though it may sometimes appear impossible, we *do* have the power to change our attitude when it is in our best interest. Laughing and appreciating the humor in our own life circumstances can help us to do just that.

It is important for children to laugh and to play. Why should it be any less important for adults: just because we have bigger bodies? Think about the ways you have fun. How often do you just relax and play? When I lead groups for women who eat compulsively, I always set aside at least one group meeting to look at the absence of fun and play in most of our lives. I instruct the women simply to play and I leave the room. When I return fifteen minutes later the women are inevitably sitting where they were when I left with bewildered expressions on their faces. Usually they are engaged in sharing their confusion about my direction. The instruction to play renders them helpless. They tell me that they don't know what "play" is supposed to mean for an adult. We talk about this and, after some encouragement, they reminisce about ways they played as children.

Do you remember how to play? Please "lighten up" and enjoy yourself more often. Rent funny movies, read humorous books, watch and listen to good comedians, tell jokes, play with the children around you and let them teach you how to keep life in perspective. Smile and laugh as often as possible! It takes fewer muscles to laugh than it does to frown, so smile more. Smile at others and then go to the mirror and smile at yourself. *The more you develop a positive attitude and notice the humor in your life, the more calm and loving you will feel and the more gently you will treat yourself. The more gently you treat yourself, the less likely you will be to feel tense and to seek relief by eating too much.* When your Chew "acts out" you will be able to understand and ignore her. You will recognize that she is part of you—that her existence is inevitable within any human being—and you will be able to think of her in a less serious way. Then you will be able to say "no" to her persistent demands. You will be truly free.

Reflections

CHAPTER IX

Healing the Social Self

AWARENESS

HOW can we begin to heal the wounds of our social development? From early on we have been taught to value youth more than age. We have been instructed to be thin, to smile, work hard, anticipate and take care of everyone's needs—to be impossibly perfect. We have all been so bombarded with messages like these that it is hard to hear our own voices above the din. It is difficult to be told what society expects us to be like and then to choose something else. We risk disapproval and fear others will disconnect from us if we behave in ways that threaten social norms. So, how do we start? You have already begun as you have read through these pages. You have been increasing your awareness and that is the most important step. Without awareness, things are confusing and mysterious. We only know we are uncomfortable. We don't feel quite right but we don't know why.

One way to develop greater awareness is to read from the many fine helping books that focus on the issues of self-image, self-esteem, body image, and empowerment. In the back of this book you will find a reading list. On it there are suggested readings that will enhance your understanding of your food compulsions from the holistic perspectives we are exploring: physical, emotional, social and spiritual. Armed with knowledge of these subjects, you will be able to question and evaluate things for yourself. You will no longer be dependent upon society and others to dictate to you. You will be free to explore who you are and to act in ways that fit you. You will no longer have to pressure yourself to fit into any mold. Your focus will shift from needing external forces to guide you to trusting your inner wisdom as you make choices and take actions. You will become fully in charge of yourself and your choices. You will then be free to make your own mistakes and to reap the rewards of your own accomplishments.

I strongly urge clients to participate in some type of group activity. Often they resist this idea at first. Women may secretly fear that others will not accept them or understand, or they may feel ashamed and embarrassed that they have problems. ("What is wrong with *me* that *I* feel out of control?") They fear going into a group and talking because they see their problems as different from everybody else's problems. ("Why am *I* eating compulsively when others *appear* to be doing so well?") There is a double standard that goes something like this: "I can understand and sympathize with someone else's struggles but *I* should not struggle in these ways. Being in a group would probably help other people but I am sure that a group experience isn't for *me*."

You may have entertained similar thoughts. If you think a group is only for someone else, you are wrong. If you think you don't need others to support you, again, you are wrong. Thinking that *you* have to be perfect when no one else does is the kind of subtle and insidious message your Chew sends you. Please reconsider your position about group support and find out what opportunities exist in your area. It is natural to feel timid or nervous at first but push yourself to attend anyway. If you feel shy, take your time and get to know people. You don't have to blurt out all of your private and personal thoughts and feelings to anyone. In fact, it is important *not* to do that. You need to set clear boundaries (remember?) and to build trust and confidence gradually.

Meeting regularly with a support group or a discussion group can help you to develop a positive and empowered self-image. You will feel less isolated, your feelings will be validated, and you will benefit by "belonging." Some women report that being in a group was the first time they had ever felt "connected"—like they fit in. In a group setting, you can allow people into your life who will get to know you, and who are likely to be there for you when you need support. Having a group of women gather to talk, to share experiences and feelings, and to raise each others' consciousness is exciting. I have facilitated many groups and I can assure you that when women convene to share their thoughts and feelings with one another, it is an adventure. Women often come into a group feeling isolated, depressed or discouraged and leave the group energized after experiencing the healing power that comes just from being in the presence of like-minded people and being heard. No, all your problems won't be solved when you leave but you might have a different perspective about them. The problems you came with remain, but you leave knowing you are not alone with them. You have talked, and people have shown you that they care by listening. This can give you the strength and courage you need to face things in your life.

Groups of any kind can be powerful vehicles for growth. We all need to feel connected and all of us benefit from the validation and support groups can provide. I strongly urge you to explore possibilities for some type of group involvement in your area. Being in volunteer or work groups can help you feel connected. Some people find this through twelve step programs like Alcoholics Anonymous or Overeaters Anonymous. If you attend meetings such as this, you may want to consider attending some all-female meetings in addition to some mixed-gender ones. (Women's issues are sometimes quite different from men's and women often report they feel self-conscious and inhibited with males present.) Some women attend reading groups or get together through churches, counseling centers, women's organizations, sports or schools, for example. Some women seek like-minded neighbors and friends and plan regular times to get together just to talk and "hang out." *No matter how you connect with women, the connecting itself is what's important. Connection empowers you to feel accepted, to grow and to change.* You will discover that others have feelings similar to yours and this can help you to feel more confident and calm and less apt to rely on binges to soothe yourself.

CHALLENGING OLD BELIEFS

As we discussed earlier, we have received many messages throughout the years about how we are to behave, to look, to dress, to eat, to be, and how we are to feel about it. These messages came and continue to come to us from many sources. Part of changing how we feel about ourselves and changing our food abusive patterns means taking a long, hard look at the messages we personally have received and challenging them. Allow yourself to feel angry about society's mandates to you to be thin, young, and perfect as judged by unrealistic standards. You need to challenge these messages if you are to disregard them. Ask yourself, "Why should I be silent? Why do I hesitate to stand up for myself and my rights as a human being? Why do I wear clothes that are constricting and uncomfortable? Why do I put other's needs way ahead of my own? Why do I do things I really don't want to do?" These and so many other questions need to be asked and thought about.

List questions to ask yourself. Think about the messages you have heard in your lifetime. Do you think you must always be "nice" to everyone around you and that you can never say "no" to others? Do you think your needs and wants don't count as much as those of others? Do you think your feelings are not as important as someone else's feelings or that you must wear a size eight dress? Do you harbor beliefs that you cannot further your education or take time for yourself to relax? Do you secretly think a man is more important, intelligent or valuable than you? Do you think you can't eat certain foods? Begin to notice areas where your thinking has been influenced by messages you have received from many sources (e.g. the media, church, government, family, peers and teachers). Let yourself dare to challenge these messages and to move past them. Make the decisions you want to make and take the actions you wish to take.

If we are to genuinely relax and enjoy the time we have on this planet, then we need to act in ways that are fitting and true for us. *As long as we try to tailor our looks, our behaviors and our feelings to the expectations of others, or the perfectionistic expectations we have internalized, we will not feel good about ourselves and we will continue sabotaging ourselves in self-destructive ways as we have in the past.* Our Chew will remain willful and strong. We will stuff ourselves with chocolate, potato chips, macaroni and cheese, or ice cream to dull our feelings. We will binge to mask the anger we feel when we fail to pay attention to our own needs. We will make "self-loathing" choices as long as we do not treat *ourselves* with the respect and consideration we give to *others*. Much of our self-destructive food behavior is a result of the negative feelings that arise when we don't attend to ourselves—when we don't make *ourselves* our top priority.

COMMUNICATION AND ASSERTIVENESS

It is one thing for a woman to challenge old beliefs and to recognize her budding desire to behave in new ways, and quite another to know how to begin. As we touched upon in the previous section on *Healing the Emotional Self,* women often find they lack the skills and the confidence necessary to implement the changes they wish to make. When we have been silent and passive a good deal of our lives, it is difficult to become clear, direct and assertive. Although we can easily see that other people are valuable and have rights, we may view ourselves as exceptions to this rule. It is often a shift in focus to begin to see ourselves as worthy, and as valuable as anyone else. This shift cannot and does not occur easily, nor does it occur over night. We may agree intellectually that all people, male or female, have certain basic human rights, but to actually recognize and stand up for these rights for ourselves is challenging. It is a challenge worth taking on, however, and essential to creating a peaceful and serene life—a life that is free of compulsive behavior.

As part of my practice I help women learn the skills they need to communicate clearly and assertively. I emphasize the importance of assertiveness and good communication skills to highlight the importance of experiencing your personal power by defining clear, unmistakable, strong boundaries in all areas of your life. Learning how to do this is absolutely necessary. *If we are to conquer our compulsive eating behaviors and feel in control of our lives, we must express ourselves fully.* This is *essential.* In the section on *Awareness* at the start of this chapter I have suggested courses or groups in which communication and assertiveness skills are taught and practiced. I run groups specifically designed so that women can learn to be direct, clear and assertive (not aggressive—that is different). Members can practice the skills they are learning within the safety of the group. They can experiment. Any new behavior feels awkward at first and it is helpful to practice with others who share the same fears and feelings of inadequacy. This helps build the confidence necessary to make changes.

By the way, just because you have decided to begin taking care of yourself and sticking up for your beliefs and feelings does not mean that those around you will necessarily be happy about it. They may even be openly disapproving of your growth and changes, at least initially. People resist change and when you start acting differently they may not appreciate it. When you begin to take yourself and your needs more seriously and to make yourself a priority, others may become fearful and feel threatened. They may wonder if you are transforming into a non-caring monster of some sort. When you stop playing the "caretaker of the universe" role, people close to you may become frightened and try to sabotage your efforts. They may not understand your changes and may fear that you will not be there for them anymore.

It takes time and patience to make lasting changes and it also takes time for those around you to adjust to and accept the "new you." As people realize that you taking care of yourself does not automatically mean harming or abandoning them, your relationships should stabilize and become more meaningful and genuine. If some people in your life cannot tolerate your changes and insist that you remain passive or that you continue to deny your needs in favor of theirs, you might ask yourself why you want to be in that relationship. You may even decide to let that particular relationship go.

Sometimes women find that some of their relationships have been built on unhealthy premises. Becoming clear, direct and assertive, however, gives you the tools you need to make necessary changes within these connections. You can talk with those who are important to you about your need to change and, if the relationship is worth working on, they will be open to hearing you and discussing any changes you both need to make. They will support you, accept you and adjust to your new ways of interacting. Hopefully, they will also ask questions and be willing to share their concerns and fears in discussions with you. When both people in any relationship share their thoughts and feelings freely with one another and each feels heard and respected, they enhance an already healthy relationship through these interactions.

As you use the skills you are learning to take control in various areas of your life, you will feel more in control of your food behaviors. This is not a coincidence. Being fully expressive and responsible for our own behaviors and feelings makes a great difference. When we speak up clearly and in an openhearted way, we feel proud of ourselves and we give ourselves the message that we count. We don't view ourselves as more or less important than anyone else. Instead we simply realize that we are equal to others. We don't speak out to control others, to belittle them, hurt them or to win power struggles. We simply state what is *our* truth. We let others know how *we* see things and how *we* feel. They may not see things our way or agree with us. That is okay. We speak with no expectation that others will agree or disagree. We are each unique beings—that's what makes this world a fascinating place. *There is great freedom in self-expression. With it comes a feeling of being alive and empowered. When we feel free in this way, stuffing ourselves with food is not a viable option.*

Reflections

CHAPTER X

Healing the Spiritual Self

WHERE TO BEGIN?

HOW do we heal our spirits? What a big question that is! Where do we begin? Who can teach us the secrets of connecting with a spiritual source or feeling within ourselves? Many of us have felt a yearning to develop this part of ourselves, but how? When? Where do we go? What do we do? This can seem foreign and even frightening if we have never explored it before. Many of us have had the feeling that there must be more to life than day-to-day struggles but have no idea what it might be. This wondering is useful and can lead us on a more meaningful path. A spiritual journey can be precipitated in any number of ways. It often begins with a vague sense of discontent. We may feel a stirring somewhere deep inside. When we pay attention to it, we become compelled to learn more about ourselves and to listen to our inner voices.

For some of us, connection with spirit follows a particularly difficult time. Clients frequently report such experiences as vital parts of their growth. In her book, *Appetites,* Geneen Roth openly shares her painful journey. A lifetime of struggle with weight, food and severe illness eventually led her on her search for spiritual growth. In another inspiring book, *Guilt is the Teacher, Love is the Lesson,* Joan Borysenko writes about her personal struggles as a young girl and how her spiritual journey began at that time. I myself can recall a number of painful experiences which seemed devastating as I was experiencing them but, when viewed in retrospect, were rich with life lessons. These painful times helped me to open my heart and my mind and to search for spiritual meaning in my life. Think about your own life and the difficult situations you have faced. Perhaps you can see how such experiences have led you to seek some kind of spiritual meaning in your life as well.

You may have noticed that many people who seem the most grounded, connected or spiritual have suffered in their lifetimes. Pain is necessary for growth and the amount of growth may be commensurate with the amount of pain. This does not mean we are required to suffer gravely in order to become spiritual. It does follow, however, that we need to struggle through difficulties at times in order to learn life lessons and to grow. It is impossible to maintain this perspective at all times. It is hard to appreciate that we are growing when we are in the midst of personal chaos. *When we are having a hard time we would do well to embrace our pain as useful and necessary for our development.*

This is not an easy lesson to learn but please remind yourself of it, if you can remember, when you are in crisis. I often share the following with clients who are in distress: Chinese people draw symbols to make their words. One character, or symbol, they make represents crisis. The identical symbol also means danger and opportunity. They recognize that any time of life crisis has within it the potential for greatest growth and opportunity. I have never seen this fail. When any of us passes through the pain of our life crises, we can emerge into a time of opportunity.

LIVING IN THE PRESENT

We spend most of our time living in either the past or the future. We are either thinking about what we have already done, perhaps with regret, or we are spinning off into the future, perhaps overwhelming ourselves. This may be human nature but it is not helpful to us when we are trying to let go of unhealthy habits and change our approach to life in general and to food control behaviors in particular.

If we allow ourselves to focus on the past, we are setting ourselves up for trouble. It is tempting to obsess about mistakes we have made and things that have gone wrong. Seldom do we concentrate on all the things we have done right or that have gone well. This is one of the many tricks of our Chew. Keeping ourselves stuck in the past ruminating about things we cannot change is futile. It is a waste of our energy and keeps us in a negative frame of mind. You can think about the whole package of Girl Scout cookies you ate until the cows come home but it won't change the fact that the cookies are gone. There is nothing you can do now about a choice you made last night. Continuing to beat yourself up about it only makes matters worse. *This is a time to remind yourself to come into the present.* Let the thoughts of cookies go and think instead about what you want for yourself in the present moment. How do you want to behave right now? How can you take the best care of yourself and get your needs met in the moment? Tell your Chew that you are not listening and to "*stop!*" Turn your energy and attention towards nurturing yourself in the present moment.

Operating in the future is as destructive as focusing on the past but in different ways. When you allow yourself to anticipate what the future holds for you, you are likely to either expect problems that may not materialize or to set yourself up with expectations that may not be met. Either way, this is another waste of precious time and energy. A third consequence of thinking too much into the future is the likelihood that you will overwhelm yourself. If you begin, for example, to think of all the things you have to do, the pending workload will seem impossible to cope with. You will be tired before you begin and you will have great difficulty moving ahead. You may instead find yourself remaining stuck and shoving chocolate, pasta or more Girl Scout cookies into your mouth. As you must do when you notice your mind is in the past, remind yourself to come back from the future into present time.

None of us can operate in present time at every moment. We probably spend 90% of our time in the past or the future. Begin to notice this in your own thought patterns. If you would like to learn more, I highly recommend you read the works of Thich Nhat Hanh, a Buddhist monk who writes beautifully about being mindful and living in the present. The teachings of this gentle man guide us in the art of being in each moment and appreciating fully our experience here on earth. He advises us to focus on the present moment as often as possible, to breathe deeply and to smile.

Thich Nhat Hanh tells us that in the community in which he lives everyone observes moments of silence regularly throughout the day. A mindfulness bell is rung at regular intervals and when each resident hears it, he or she stops what they are doing for a moment to breathe, to smile and to remind themselves to be in the present moment. If you have a watch equipped with an alarm, set it to signal you each hour. When your alarm sounds, do as Thich Nhat Hanh suggests: breathe, smile and remind yourself to be in the present moment.

If we fail to focus on the present and allow our energy and attention to jump back and forth between past and future, we lose the present. In doing so, we miss opportunities to feel and experience our lives. This behavior keeps us eating, and eating even more, in an effort to feel satisfied and alive. Eating, of course, doesn't help. If we are out of touch with our feelings and experiences in the present, we will continue the pattern of overeating. We will beat ourselves up emotionally and then eat even more. We will notice that time is passing by while we are sitting on the side lines observing life instead of living it. *When you notice that you are in past or future time, remind yourself to return to the present. The past is gone and the future is not yet here to command your attention. You need all of your energy to be here now.*

THE IMPORTANCE OF ENVIRONMENT

When we are eating in an "out of control" way, it generally means we are feeling out of control in other areas of our lives as well. Often these chaotic feelings are reflected in our environment. We are exposed to crime and violence each day in our culture. In his best selling book, *Eight Weeks to Optimum Health,* Andrew Weil, M.D. recommends we do a "news fast" periodically. This is great advice. Giving yourself a break from the trauma in the world gives you a chance to recover from its upsetting effects. Try this one day per week or more.

I would like to take a few minutes here to reflect on environment in three different ways. Let's consider the environment we create for ourselves indoors, the environment nature provides for us outdoors and the environment we harbor deep within ourselves. All of these are important to think about and attend to. If we do not feel peaceful in our surroundings it is very hard to feel peaceful within ourselves. Our feelings are reflected in our environment and vice versa.

Sometimes, when we are feeling off-center, attending to our various environments can help us to feel better.

First, think about the indoor places where you spend time. Consider not only your home but your work environment as well. Do you feel peaceful in these settings? Are they furnished and decorated in ways that are conducive to relaxation or do they reflect the chaos you may be experiencing? Take a look around and ask yourself, "What can I do in this setting to create an environment where I can really relax?" Now, I am not talking here about throwing out all your old furniture and overspending your credit cards redecorating. This isn't about spending money. This is about creating peaceful space.

Recently my son and daughter-in-law realized that their environment was not conducive to relaxation. They operate on a fairly tight budget and so any major changes were out of the question. First they looked around to see what items were truly important to them and what things were not. Next they identified those items that were unnecessary and could be eliminated. Then they reorganized what they chose to keep and spent time thoroughly cleaning their space. They began playing classical music softly and occasionally burning wonderfully aromatic incense or candles. With very little money, but much creativity and enthusiasm, they changed the whole atmosphere of their home. Instead of coming home in the evening to a disorganized, crowded place, they truly made their home a refuge that they looked forward to entering after long hours of tiring work.

Look around your work and living spaces and, if you are dissatisfied with them, ask yourself what you can do to change the feeling of the space. Fresh flowers on your desk at the office can make a world of difference. Music can relax or energize you. A tiny crystal hanging in a sunny window will fill your space with dancing rainbows and invite joy. A picture of a peaceful scene can improve your mood. Sometimes just cleaning and organizing can change your whole outlook. When we get frantic about things or feel depressed or anxious, these uncomfortable feelings do get reflected in the spaces we occupy. It is all connected. If we overlook the importance of a peaceful external environment, we set ourselves up to create a chaotic environment within ourselves. Our environment reflects us as we, in turn, reflect it. So take a few minutes to look around and become aware. Create a feeling on the outside that you would like to experience inside.

To help you in your effort to maximize the pleasure you can find in your environment, I recommend you read Kathryn Terah Collins book, *The Western Guide to Feng Shui* (pronounced "fung shway"). In this exciting book, Ms Collins explains this oriental practice. She teaches that life force or energy, known as "Chi" energy, flows all around us and that by arranging our homes and work and play areas in certain ways we increase the flow of this vital "Chi" energy. This reorganization of energies creates more relaxing and energizing spaces within our existing homes. The book is worth reading and the techniques worth experimenting with. I (and others I know) have incorporated some of the principles of Feng Shui into our homes. Not only did we have fun doing this but we all noticed a definite increase of positive energy. Try it for yourself and see.

Next, observe your outdoor environment. Look at where you live. Do you notice any odors? Do you smell flowers or autumn leaves or the ocean? Can you see the color of the sky? If you live in a high rise building do you ever go out onto the roof? Do you spend a few minutes in the sunshine and in nature each day? If you live in the city, do you take time away to hike or go to the beach or just to walk down a country road? We are all a part of something larger. We are all a part of our mother earth and it is healing to be close to her as often as possible. I cannot stress strongly enough the importance of tuning-in to all the wonder nature has to offer. If we are to feel content and set aside our drive for food, we need to nourish ourselves in other ways. We are a society on the go and seldom do most of us take the time to really experience and appreciate our surroundings.

I had a magnificent opportunity to experience nature during my passage into my fiftieth year of life. As the time of my birthday approached, I decided I wanted to do something extraordinary to celebrate this awesome transition. I contacted a group based in Sausalito, California called *Wilderness Transitions* and joined with them to experience a four-day vision quest. For those of you who have not heard of such a thing, I must tell you that it is a beautiful and powerful experience. We "vision questers" were taught about the environment we would be in and about first aid and safety issues by our two competent leaders (both female, by the way) during several meetings prior to our actual trip. Then we all went into the desert near Death Valley and explored the area in pairs to find remote, individual campsites. The next morning each of us set out alone to make camp at the sight we had chosen the day before.

We had a check system in place so that if one of us were to become ill or to be injured, someone would come to us. If not, we would be on our own for four days and nights and no one would come near. During this time, we would abstain from food entirely and cleanse our bodies with a gallon of water per day, herbal teas and a mixture of lemon juice, cayenne pepper and maple syrup. During this experience, I had the time to sit still in nature and to observe plants and animals in a way that I never had before. We do not and cannot ordinarily spend this much time idle, having nothing more to do than watch a sunset.

Prior to the trip I had considered myself fairly attuned to nature, but I came home from Death Valley knowing I am not just an observer of nature. I am as much a part of it as the grandest tree or the tiniest pebble. To sit for hours in silence on a rock watching flowers move gently in a breeze or a lizard sunning herself on a rock can be a remarkable adventure. I experienced a peace during my quest that is hard to describe. I simply sat, breathed and allowed myself to tune in to the sights, sounds and smells all around me. I never gave one thought to food. It was not important. I was completely nourished by the beauty of nature that enveloped me.

Most people never have an opportunity to walk off into the desert alone for four days and many people would not care to do that even if they had the chance. You do not need to fast, however and spend days alone to tune in to the earth. Just get out into nature and let yourself absorb the experience with all of your senses. Notice the sun as it rises and sets each day. Close your eyes and focus on the sounds and smells around you. If you can't get away often, bring a bit of the outdoors inside. Add seashells, feathers, interesting rocks, branches and plants to your home or office. Put a tiny indoor fountain in your space. Bring nature into your environment and then set aside a few minutes every day to appreciate and enjoy it.

Attend to your internal environment as well. Spend time sitting still, listening to your breath and the sounds around you. Begin to think of yourself as "spirit"—connected to universal energy. If you are religious, connect with others of your faith. Meditate. Work on developing an attitude of love and gratitude. Be gentle with yourself. Remind yourself that there are no mistakes—only lessons. Write in your journal. Paint. Read interesting and inspiring books. Listen to music. Observe animals. Pet them. Play with them. Spend time with children. Laugh every time you have a chance (and make chances often). Surround yourself with beauty and give yourself the solitude in which to enjoy it. We all need quiet time. We need to breathe and to reflect. *We all need time to go within and to listen to our own voices. Only then can we hear the words of wisdom that we all have deep within our core selves. We are all connected to the earth and remembering that each day can help us feel vibrant and relaxed. Then we can appreciate our spiritual selves and only then can we end our urges to abuse ourselves with food.*

WORKING WITH THE PAIN

All of us have endured pain in some way during our lifetimes. Many of us have been sexually, physically or emotionally abused. Many of us have felt abandoned in our lives. Some of us may have received negative messages about ourselves and about our worth from very early on. These are all terrible injuries and very painful. There is "old" pain from our childhood to move through and "new" pain that comes along throughout our lives. If we suffer an injury or illness, this is pain. If we lose a loved one or watch them suffer, this is pain and when we end a destructive relationship or fail an exam, this is pain too.

Earlier I referred to pain as opportunity for growth but sometimes the growth accompanying the pain comes well disguised. We may feel depressed or anxious and not know where these feelings are coming from or what growth might come through them. Let me share an example from my own life. Many years ago a woman I knew felt badly hurt by me. Instead of confronting me directly, she decided to complain about me to others and soon many other women in the area heard of her story. Although her story contained threads of truth, the information that I became aware of was largely exaggerated and false. I felt helpless to stop the gossip and to put an end to the hurtful talk. Rumors flew for a while and I had no chance to correct any of the misinformation that was circulating. No one talked with me about the stories they were hearing and I had no opportunities to defend myself. No one asked to hear my side of the story and I lost many relationships with women I had cared for and thought of as my friends. People that I had trusted and shared my life experiences and feelings with suddenly ended our friendships. I felt helpless, victimized, abandoned, out of control, bewildered, lost and betrayed (to name just a few of my feelings).

For a long time (years, actually) I felt "bad." My self-esteem was badly damaged and, even though I had never intended to hurt anyone,

I began to see myself as a "bad" person. I abandoned myself. I went from feeling connected and vital to this community of women to being viewed and treated as an outcast. Sometimes I felt victimized and harassed. Sometimes I felt mad at the women who complained and gossiped about me. At other times I felt abandoned and terribly lonely and sad. I went through a staggering range of emotions over and over and over again. I became obsessed with these feelings and the situation and, long after the situation was over and the rumors had ceased, I remained obsessed with it. I beat myself up and cried and ate and felt utterly horrible and ate more. It was a time of great darkness for me. I couldn't see even a glimmer of light at the end of the tunnel. I couldn't find anything positive about the situation. If the amount of my growth was to match the intensity of my pain, I thought, then I should be growing like a weed. But I didn't feel any of the exhilaration of growth. Instead I felt only the frustration of being stuck and alienated.

The way out of negativity came gradually. I meditated and nurtured myself as much as I could. I wrote pages and pages in my journal. I vented my feelings and then tried to sit still and listen to the voices deep inside myself for guidance. I read beautiful books about spirit and I went to talk with a spiritual guide on a few occasions. I spent some weekends at a retreat center (called Kripalu) in Lenox, Massachusetts. There I practiced yoga daily, ate healthy food, sometimes cried, walked, wrote in my journal and reflected quietly on my past and on the upsetting situation at hand. I had always been interested in spiritual matters but the painful events from which I was recovering speeded me along my spiritual journey. The chaos of the situation provided questions, and silent reflection eventually brought answers. Now I can honestly say that I feel grateful for having had that experience. At the time I never thought I would see it in this way, but I do.

In hindsight, I thank these women for treating me in the ways they did. It was unfair, hurtful and traumatic. It was surely one of the hardest times I have ever had and I would not ever want to go through it again. In retrospect, however, it did provide the richest of life lessons. I learned from it all to have crystal clear boundaries with people and to speak out when things do not seem fair or just. I learned to be more thoughtful, less impulsive and to be patient with myself and others when we make mistakes (as we all do). I learned to nurture and appreciate the loving relationships I have with others and to attend to my relationship with myself. I think I am more understanding and tolerant as a result and I am able to feel good about myself and my behavior most of the time.

In complicated situations I am able to see more of the picture—never to consider one person's perspective as the whole story. I feel more confident and solid and I learned that, even though people may disconnect from me, I do not need to disconnect from *myself.* I can go inside now to seek the truth and the consolation I had previously depended on others to provide. I am stronger and more in touch with loving myself. I feel lighter, happier, more spiritual, more connected —all this from such a difficult, painful experience!

It is hard to step aside for a moment when you are in pain to remind yourself that it will pass and that you will be stronger and wiser for having gone through it. When things are difficult, learn to go within yourself to find the answers you need and to heal. Write in your journal, take walks in nature and use your support system. Let your emotions flow freely. Cry. Stamp your feet. Express yourself. Meditate. Think about your situation and about what you can do realistically to change things. Do what you can and let the rest go. Remind yourself that there are life lessons in all your experiences and think about what life lessons may be found in your current upsetting situation. Turn to your own spiritual or religious beliefs. Pray for guidance and acceptance if prayer is part of your belief system. *When things seem the darkest for you, realize that there are lessons in the situation and you are learning and growing. You don't have to like the situation or the pain to work on accepting it. The less you resist it the more quickly it will pass and the less likely you will be to eat your way through it.*

Reflections

Part III

Pulling It All Together— Where We Go from Here

MAKING SELF-LOVING CHOICES

O NCE I went to visit a friend of mine and I noticed that she had taped several signs up in various places around her home. She had one next to her old-fashioned, claw-foot bathtub, another next to the full-length mirror in her bedroom, one over the kitchen sink, another in her study. Each sign was colorful. She had used many shades of watercolor paint and each had a little scene on it, such as the sun rising over a mountain, or a few tiny pine trees decorating a corner. Imprinted on each sign was the question, "Is this a self-loving choice?" I asked my friend about these signs. She laughed and started to say something about having forgotten their presence and that I must think her a little nuts. . . I assured her that I didn't and exclaimed that I loved the message. She explained to me that she was learning to make self-loving choices for herself at the time. These signs, she explained, served as visual cues to help her get into the habit of asking herself that question. They helped her to get the message into her conscious and subconscious minds.

143

One concept central to the business of taking care of ourselves is the idea of making as many self-loving choices as we can, as often as we can. Throughout this book we have looked closely at the behavior of compulsive eating. We have examined the issue from physical, emotional, spiritual and social perspectives to empower ourselves with knowledge. We have considered ways we can begin making changes in our lifestyles to accommodate our new ways of thinking about our bodies and food. One way to attend to the whole picture at once is to think in terms of consistently making as many self-loving choices in each area as we can.

For most of us it is easier to be as conscious as possible about each food choice than it is to measure food or count calories or track the grams of fat we consume. Also, this weighing, measuring, or counting can keep us focused on our weight whereas developing a "habit" of making self-loving choices is a way to lose weight that works slowly, but effectively, over the long term. When I suggest this, however, I do so with a bit of caution. It can be tempting to think that whatever we want is a self-loving choice. For example, it may be tempting to think, "That cookie looks good. I love cookies. I would be happy eating it. Doing something that makes me happy is a self-loving choice; Therefore, eating that cookie would be a self-loving choice." WRONG. Unless:

1. you have made a decision that you will feel resentful and deprived without that cookie and
2. you are making a conscious choice to eat that cookie and
3. you know that it is likely to set you up for sugar cravings and
4. you plan to take care of yourself in some way when cravings do follow and
5. you promise not to punish yourself after for having eaten it.

If you try to fool yourself by rationalizing and you don't think your choices through, then you set yourself up for failure and frustration. This type of faulty thinking is a trap. It is your Chew trying to trick you. Tell her to take a hike. Sit down. Take a deep breath and evaluate the situation. After you think it through, you can choose to eat the cookie or not, but your choice will be a conscious one, well thought-out and made with an attitude of love.

Most of us would agree that choosing a piece of fruit instead of a chocolate bar is obviously a self-loving choice. I believe that instinctively each of us knows what our bodies really need nutritionally. Deep inside we really do know what our needs are. From the time of our birth, however, we have been discouraged from trusting ourselves about what we eat. Our parents, teachers, television commercials, diet authorities, and magazines all dictate to us what we should choose. We may try to "do it right" and please others, so we listen to all these messages and become more confused and out of touch with ourselves than ever.

I am suggesting here that there is a different way to think and act, a healthier way. Coming from our own place of power and knowledge, we can ask ourselves continually if something we are about to do is a self-loving choice. This applies to the decisions we make about what we put into our mouths and also to any choices we face as we negotiate our way through each moment in time. We know it is self-loving to relax at times and at other times to go for a walk or a brisk run. It is self-loving to say "no" to others at times and to maintain clear boundaries for ourselves.

Self-loving choices come in many different forms. It is self-loving, for example, to wear warm clothing in cold weather, to take quiet time and space regularly, to drink cool, clear, non-chlorinated water, to brush our teeth, and to give ourselves attention. Some self-loving choices are obvious and are easy to make. Others are difficult to recognize and to follow through with. Sometimes we do something or eat something that is not in our best interest. Afterwards, we see that we might have made a better choice. *Making self-loving choices continuously may be our intention, actually doing so every time is impossible.* Perfection is not the goal. It is instead to become increasingly aware that you do have the power of choice and to use that power to make self-loving choices as often as you can in every area of your life. This is difficult at first but it does get easier with practice. Making self-loving choices is self-reinforcing. As you make a healthy choice and notice that you feel good about it, you will want to make more self-loving choices and to feel even better.

A few months following my trip to my friend's house and my discovery of her signs, I returned for another visit. Apparently her strategy for change was effective because her old signs had been replaced by new ones. Each was large and had printed upon it in bold red magic marker the exclamation, "I make self-loving choices!"

MANAGING STRESS

Stress is part of our everyday life. We can't get around it. It is necessary for our survival. We need to feel stressed at times to perform optimally. Sometimes, however, stress in our fast-pace, high-tech world can be negative and its effects are detrimental to our peace of mind and our health. We must do what we can to avoid this type of stress but we cannot escape it entirely. When we are stressed, an avalanche of feelings accompanies that state. Eating is a way many of us have learned to calm ourselves and quiet the din of voices inside. One major reason for overeating is to calm stressed-out feelings. It is necessary to understand this and to practice different ways to deal with our stresses if we are to stop eating compulsively once and for all.

An effective stress management program should include as many of the following as possible:

- eating a healthy diet of fresh, whole, natural foods (including plenty of non-chlorinated water).
- making sure that you get plenty of rest.
- developing an exercise plan tailored to your needs (both aerobic exercise and stretching).
- letting go of perfectionistic self-expectations.
- suspending harsh judgements of others as well as of yourself.
- intentionally developing a positive attitude.
- meditating, or regularly practicing an activity which incorporates deep breathing and silence.
- spending ample time in nature to remind you of your connection to the earth and to spirit.
- spending time alone to acknowledge and experience your feelings.
- communicating your feelings respectfully, assertively and lovingly.
- stimulating yourself intellectually from time to time.
- expressing yourself creatively—music, dance, art, theater, writing, gardening, etc.
- using and appreciating your support system.
- enriching your personal connections by attending to relationships in your life.

– seeing the humor in situations as often as you can.

– keeping your living environment pleasant and relaxing.

– living as mindfully as possible in present time.

Do these things as frequently as you can. Develop a stress plan for yourself. Copy the preceding list of ways you can combat stress and put it where you can refer to it often. It will serve as a reminder to attend to yourself in many different ways. I encourage you to take a few minutes each day to ask yourself how *you* are doing. All day long we greet people by asking, "How are you today?" Do we take the time to ask, "How am *I* today?" When was the last time you actually took the time to sit down quietly and check in with yourself? *Because life is so full of distractions, we need to remind ourselves again and again and again to make ourselves our number one priority. We must nurture ourselves often and in as many ways as we can—physically, emotionally, socially and spiritually.* Your Chew will balk when you attempt to do this. Don't listen. Persevere in your efforts to love and care for yourself. Your reward for doing so will be inner peace, self-control and increased self-esteem.

THE BOARD MEETING

Have you ever been in a corporation or group of some kind run by a Board of Directors? Directors sit on Boards which oversee the workings of all the facets of an organization and they must meet often and regularly to do so. Well, this idea can be helpful for personal use too. This is how it works. Either by yourself or with a friend or two, plan a time when you will hold your board meetings. It is best to set regular times, such as every other Friday morning, for example. Next think of all the committees you will want to have report on their activity. You may have a work committee, a rest committee, eating committee, stress management committee, exercise committee, etc. Make a list of these committees and then either by yourself, or with others, take one committee (one area of your life) at a time and reflect upon it. Take time to pay attention to each of your committees to see if they have been operating optimally or if they have been either too active or not active enough. If you are doing this with others, listen as each person reports on how each part of their organization is operating.

You may notice that your work committee has been doing a bit too much overtime and that your rest and play committees have little activity to report. You might find that your exercise committee has been totally inactive and your eating committee has overspent its budget and gone wild. Board meetings provide structure which can be a useful way to keep tabs on yourself. We are all so busy with the business of getting through life that we can get easily out of balance and not even realize it. Regular board meetings can help us keep on track. It is a way to help maintain a healthy balance in all areas of life.

Also, if you plan to do this with a few friends, you will receive feedback and you can help one another not only by listening but also by offering each other suggestions for coming into and maintaining balance. You will also have the added benefit of the fun and support of regular connection. It takes a bit of planning to set this up initially, but some women I know have used it and found it very helpful. They may stick to their format or, at times, they may end up discussing how they are doing in less formal ways. However they handle their gatherings, they usually report that they end up feeling better just because they took the time to connect with others and to think about how they have been taking care of themselves (or not taking care of themselves).

When committees report to the Board, they evaluate their level of activity and modify this activity to best serve the company. If a committee has been active, conscientious and balanced, the company benefits as a result. You benefit when your committees are active and balanced as well. If all of your committees are engaging in an appropriate amount of activity—not over- or under-achieving—you will feel balanced. If you are exercising moderately, eating well, resting and nurturing yourself you will feel better and are less likely to overeat. You must check on all these aspects of self-care, and one effective way to pay attention is to have each committee issue a "report" regularly. Your committee chairpersons *must* report periodically to ensure that all of your committees are active and working together and in your best interest.

AVOIDING A BINGE

When you feel like eating everything you can get your hands on it is difficult to stop and think about anything else but food. It is difficult at best—and at times feels impossible—to pause and reflect about your feelings and to somehow contain those powerful urges to binge. One strategy that can often help is to postpone eating for a short while. There are other options you may choose rather than overeating at that particular time. The idea is not to fight the urges you are having but instead to tell yourself you may proceed with your binge, but first you are taking at least ten to fifteen minutes to do something else. If, after these minutes have passed, you still feel like soothing yourself with food, you can make that choice. Just remember not to beat yourself up afterwards.

It is useful to make and set aside a list of things you enjoy doing. *When the urge to binge strikes tell your Chew you will make a choice to eat or not to eat only after you have done one of the activities on your list.* Then read your list. Choose one activity that you enjoy and do it. (you *may* have to *force* yourself to begin as the compulsion to binge is overwhelming at times.) Often the urges to eat are long gone by the time you are through with your diverting activity and you can go about your day feeling peaceful and happy with yourself for bypassing a binge. Following is a short sample list. Please feel free to use it as a guide, but add to it. Think about things you really enjoy and make your personal list of activities to grab when the urges threaten to overwhelm you.

For example:
- lock the bathroom door, take a hot soak, with fragrant oil, candlelight, music, cool juice to sip.
- take a walk or bicycle ride.
- set a timer and lose yourself in a novel for 20 minutes or so.
- call a friend to break isolation, to chat and get support.
- involve yourself in a project—like knitting, crocheting, etc.
- use your creative self—paint, draw, scribble, mold clay.
- meditate or pray.
- enjoy sexual release—alone or with a partner.
- make a list of things you are happy about or grateful for.
- express yourself through dance—turn on any kind of music and move.
- spend time writing in your journal—whatever comes to mind— writing anything is a great release.
- take a power nap (at times we eat because we are tired—a brief nap may be what is really needed).

– whether it is day or evening, put on your coat, step outside and look at the sky for a few moments while breathing deeply.
– sit quietly and sip a cup of hot water with lemon and honey (this often removes the craving for sweets).

Whatever you choose, the idea is to break the pattern of mindless eating. Give yourself time to breathe. Be creative. Relax, exercise, have fun and then re-evaluate your need to binge. You will often find that you feel good about yourself for making this effort and the powerful urge to eat has subsided. At other times you will still feel the urge to eat but it may not be quite as strong and you may be able to resist it. You can always continue the activity you were doing or choose another activity from your list to further postpone a binge. Usually at that point you will feel in control and the urges will have subsided. If not, however, and you choose to eat, please take a minute to decide what you will have. Choose your behavior and make a plan to take care of yourself in the aftermath. Remember, no matter what, *do not* punish yourself for choosing to take care of yourself with food this one time. At other times you can and will choose different ways to behave. No one is perfect and we all make less than self-loving choices at times. Occasionally your Chew is bound to win. This is true for all of us.

POSITIVE AND NEGATIVE SPINNING

In this illustration you can see a circle with arrows pointing in one direction. Look at this circle and visualize it as a wheel in motion with one category leading into the next. Imagine that the circle pictured here is moving in a positive direction. When this positive energy flow is going on within us, our self-esteem level is high. We are most likely then to make healthy food choices, to exercise and to relax. Our body image improves as does the quality of our relationships. We feel accepting and respectful of ourselves and others and are likely to be more assertive and communicative. As we express ourselves more, we feel more connected and positive. This improves our attitude in general and leads to greater self-confidence. We are able to take life a little less seriously and to play and have fun. All of this in turn builds self-esteem and the circle spins and repeats and reinforces itself.

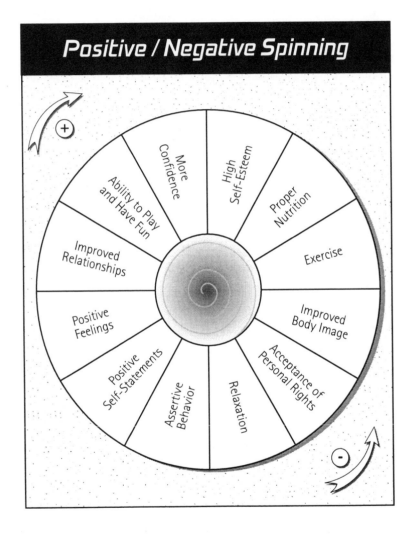

Women report that this spinning is accurate to their experience, and that all of these areas of their lives seem to move in either a completely positive direction or a completely negative one. They also report that when moving in a positive direction, the spin of the wheel can suddenly shift direction (seemingly for no reason) and just as quickly move in a negative one. When this occurs, our self-esteem suffers. When our energy begins to move in this negative direction, we are likely to behave in self-destructive ways. We make poor food choices, stop exercising and grow tense and irritable. We can't relax and our body image distorts. Our attitudes reflect our negative feelings and our relationships become strained. We lose self-respect and stop communicating. We become out of touch with our creative, playful self and our self-esteem suffers as a consequence. The negative spin then reinforces and repeats itself, just as the positive does when our wheel is spinning in a positive direction.

Many clients and friends have told me that they find it helpful to see food abusive behavior laid out in this fashion. It demystifies their experience and offers them a frame of reference from which they can make sense of their compulsive eating. Having this simple and clear illustration also provides a concrete way to look at, talk about and understand compulsive eating. Women also report that it is helpful to know that they are not alone—that their experience parallels the experience of many others.

This illustration also is a useful tool to help you change the direction of your "spinning" from a negative to a positive direction. When you begin to feel "out of control" and realize that you are spinning in a negative direction, look at the various areas included in the circle. Choose as many as possible to impact upon and you will change the direction of your spinning motion from a negative direction to a positive one. For example, if you are eating compulsively and feeling badly about yourself, you can make a decision to do concrete things to help yourself. You might go for a run and/or do twenty minutes of yoga. You could meditate, call a friend and prepare something healthy to eat. You might take a short nap and spend a bit of time on a creative project you have been meaning to attend to. You can remind yourself to think positively and go to see an uplifting or comedic movie. The point is to take action. *When you least feel like acting—when you feel helpless, ashamed, frustrated, alone, unhappy, anxious, etc.—is the most important time to show yourself and your Chew that you are in control.* So try using the illustration to help you focus and initiate changes in areas where you feel comfortable making changes. Begin by choosing at least one area and taking an action. If you can, choose more than one area (all the better). The more areas you impact upon simultaneously, the greater your chances of turning things around.

It is not always necessary or useful to focus on reasons why you got "out of control" in the first place. If you know why your behavior ran amok, that's fine. Then you can resolve to behave differently in the future to avoid repeating a pattern of self-destructive behavior. Sometimes, however, trying to figure out why we are eating compulsively at any particular time may be a clever ploy of our Chew—a way to avoid taking constructive action. Look at the cycle. Take your actions first and later, if you care to, you can revisit the situation. In retrospect you may have more success finding the causes for your tailspin. Also remember that sometimes we cannot figure out why we behaved as we did. Then it is prudent to simply acknowledge that we experienced a difficult time and to move on. *If you beat yourself up for past behavior you will reinforce your negative self-concept and assure that your wheel will keep spinning in a negative direction.*

NO MISTAKES, ONLY LESSONS

When thinking about how to design your own plan for dealing with your compulsive eating, it is necessary to think in terms of learning, not judging. None of us is perfect (How many times have I said this?). I have often worked with women who understand this premise in regards to others but insist that they are exceptions. There are *no* exceptions. As you proceed with your life, and experiment with different ways of nurturing yourself, you will make choices at times that you will later wish you had not made. This is the human way to learn.

When you choose something that is not self-loving (like choosing to eat junk food), you may be tempted to start beating yourself up about it. If you berate yourself, put yourself down or promise yourself you will *never* do it again, you are setting yourself up to fail. By behaving this way, you are lowering your self-esteem, creating anxiety and assuring that you will act out even more next time the urge to binge arrives. Although you know you feel unhappy about having eaten junk food all day, it is *not* helpful to compound your misery by punishing yourself after.

I would like you to try an experiment. Next time you realize that you have eaten things that are not healthy for you (and we *all* do on occasion) please take a moment to focus on yourself. Find a quiet place. Sit down. Close your eyes and take a few deep breaths. First use your "nurturing parent" voice to soothe yourself, to reassure yourself that you are lovable always. If tears come, cry. Be with your feelings for a bit. Next, please talk to yourself in your self-loving "adult" voice and say something like this, "Okay, I did eat too much _____ (fill in the blank), but that doesn't mean I am a bad person. I am a good person who overate on this one occasion. I am human and I didn't make the most self-loving choice this particular time. Instead of beating myself up about it, I wonder what I can learn from it about myself. What might I learn that can help me make a different choice next time? I will use each time I overeat as an opportunity to learn more about myself. I remember, there are no mistakes, only lessons. I will be gentle with myself now and move forward."

It is helpful to cultivate an attitude of curiosity about yourself and your behavior. Welcome each "mistake" as a lesson—a chance to grow. Please be in the present as much as possible. Let things go and move on. Do not dwell on the junk food you chose. Notice instead how you felt physically and emotionally when you ate it. Learn from that. Think about what you might do differently next time and *please* nurture yourself. This is one of the most important overriding principles of all when it comes to stopping compulsive eating and taming your Chew. *There really are no mistakes, only lessons.*

Reflections

Part IV

Summing It All Up

COMMITMENT TO YOURSELF

YOU can gather all the information available on compulsive eating issues. You can become an expert on exercise and nutrition. You can earn doctoral degrees in medicine, psychology and sociology. You can have board meetings with yourself, start support groups and try all of the ideas in this book. You can follow all of the suggestions and change your eating habits, but *none of this will be effective without a sincere commitment on your part.* I am not speaking of commitment to a new exercise or diet plan, but of a much more basic and meaningful idea of commitment. I am referring to the absolute necessity of making a commitment to self. This means giving yourself what you really need and treating yourself as top priority.

Many of us grew up with the notion that others' needs were always more important than ours. Some of us learned we were not supposed to have any needs at all. So, when I speak of making ourselves and our needs number one, you may have to stretch your imagination at first to entertain this idea. It may feel uncomfortable and foreign. Let's think about this together. If we make external changes but disregard our internal needs, we will not feel satisfied or happy. Trying to fit into any mold for approval or gratification leads to resentment and anxiety. Being true to ourselves is essential and, to do this, we must think of ourselves as worthy of our own time and our own attention.

We all experience some variation of the following experience—at birth we are truly in touch with ourselves as "spirits." We know that we are positive and beautiful. We know we are perfect. We experience our "essence," so to speak, as radiant and wonderful. Unfortunately, it does not take long to lose that wondrous sense of *self as spirit.* If you observe a tiny baby you will see that she quickly begins responding to her environment. She learns about herself through her interactions with the people and things around her. Soon she learns that she must behave in certain ways to get favorable reactions. Her behavior is shaped early on. Day by day, this tiny girl becomes less in touch with herself and her spirit and more in touch with the feelings and expectations of those around her. She learns to do things for approval and loses touch with her inner voice. Her experience is our experience. We all learn to "be" as other forces shape us to be and lose sight of simply "being" ourselves. At that point, we have forgotten that we are radiant, energetic spirits.

A most important part of healing and being peaceful *at any body weight,* is getting back in touch with our spirit and learning to recognize and listen to our inner voices once again. Making a firm commitment to spending time every day doing something concrete to nurture our spiritual selves is essential. This helps us regain connection with our spirit. Taking time to turn inward leads us back to ourselves —back to remembering our perfect, sparkling, spiritual selves. In their best selling book *Make the Connection,* Bob Greene and Oprah Winfrey suggest we spend some time each day discovering something about ourselves. This is excellent advice. Ten or fifteen minutes each day of meditation, yoga, journaling or prayer, for example, can help us to stay in touch with ourselves as energetic, loving beings. This practice provides regular time for reflection which is vital to stopping compulsive behavior. There is much more to each of us than only our bodies, or the roles we play in the world. If we commit firmly to taking the time to *honor our inner selves* every day, it will make all the difference in the ways we take care of ourselves. When we pause during our hectic schedules and remind ourselves that we are more than caretakers, workers, etc. we affirm our beautiful, loving existence. Making this commitment to ourselves is primary if we are to nurture our spirits as well as our bodies.

We cannot truly nurture our bodies if we fail to attend to our spirit. Many of us have spent years looking outside of ourselves for direction. We have tried in so many ways to do what the outside world is telling us to do. We have worked hard at trying to match up to what the world has told us we must look like. Now it is time to stop. If you truly want to relax around food and feel peaceful in your life, you must turn inward to find out what you *really* want for yourself and what *really* makes you happy. If you look outside of yourself to find out how to be, you will never be true to yourself. You will always be fighting against your own nature and trying to please someone else. If you learn to be still and to listen to the voices of wisdom within your heart, you will be free. You will not be filled with resentment and frustration. Instead, you will begin to develop a plan for yourself that works for you. You will begin to eat the way you want, dress the way you feel comfortable and make life choices that are well thought-out and self-loving.

You will, of course, not be able to do this consistently at every moment. Life is not like that, as you have found out, I'm sure. *The goal is to be internally directed and to be as patient and gentle with yourself as you possibly can be.* When you feel frustrated, sad, angry . . . let yourself experience these feelings. They will pass. Tell yourself that food will only anesthetize you temporarily. Let yourself be with your feelings for a time and then move on. When you realize that your focus is outside of yourself and on everyone else, go back inside for a few moments. Remind yourself that you are a loving spirit. Give yourself a bit of space and time to nurture yourself. Communicate clearly. Be assertive. Set appropriate boundaries. Express yourself. Laugh. Play. You will find that as you allow yourself to experience your own loving energy more often, you will need outside approval less. So please attend to your real needs. Journey within and think about ways to keep your focus on yourself. Then make a commitment to incorporating these practices into your life. *Do something every day to remind yourself that you are responsible for yourself and your choices and that you are a loving, precious being. This practice will set you free from the prison of compulsive eating and you will have Tamed your Chew!*

Reflections

Concepts to Remember

FOLLOWING is a list of some salient points that I have excerpted from various sections of this book. Use this section as a quick, easy way to remind yourself of the important points you have read. Reviewing these concepts often will help you keep these ideas actively in the forefront of your mind. Please don't put this book back on the shelf and forget about it—review it often. Use the following pages to help you, especially when you notice old, self-destructive impulses beginning to surface. Often we read articles or books and find them helpful but, as time passes, we forget some of the most vital messages. Review this section regularly—at least once a month. In between, pick this book up and browse through this section any time you feel alone, frustrated or possessed by urges to eat. A few minutes revisiting this section can renew the whole book for you, help you move through these urges without acting on them, and bypass a binge. The act of doing this will also help you renew your commitment to yourself and your health.

As you read this final section, circle or highlight any concepts that are particularly meaningful for you. Doing this now will help you later when you feel a strong compulsion to eat. At that time, you will most likely not have the patience to read through this rather lengthy list, but you may find that reviewing only the items you highlighted will be a manageable task. So keep this nearby and use it often. If you are aware that you eat to excess in certain places (e.g. at work, in your car), make copies of this list and store one in each location so you can put your hands on it in a hurry. We all know how powerful these urges to feed ourselves can be and this list will be of no use if it is not easy to grab. So, when the Chew has a forceful grip on you, take a break. Breathe deeply and review the concepts that are meaningful for you. By performing this act you will pull yourself through those hard times and you will have *Tamed your Chew* once again.

CONCEPTS

Feeling out of control with food generally means you are feeling out of control in other areas of your life as well.

One reason you may eat in an "out-of-control" way is because you cannot control the experiences and feelings of those around you. Feeling out of control means feeling anxious, and *anxiety in any form will lead the way to fats and sugar in a heartbeat.*

Be aware that, whenever you are involved in any process of growth and change, urges to binge may be particularly strong.

Your feelings are interwoven with your eating behaviors but you don't need to use food to manage your feelings.

It is possible to feel under control even in the most food-focused situations.

You may be using food to reward yourself or to punish yourself. If you realize your tendency to do this, you can consciously decide whether you really want to eat or not and you will not be compelled to act on these impulses.

You know instinctively that successful weight loss and maintenance depends upon understanding and resolving feelings that you have been avoiding by numbing yourself with food.

Cravings are messages to you about how you *really* feel and what you *really* need. Pay attention to and accept your feelings. This is essential in cultivating healthy eating behavior. Your job is to pay attention to what messages these cravings are delivering to you and to give yourself what you *really* need at the time (which is most likely *not* food).

Being overweight is not simple and generally there are at least a few hidden agendas behind your eating behavior.

Once you become aware of ways you have been using food thoughtlessly, you will become more conscious. Then you will be free to make different choices.

Moving your body is necessary if you are to permanently stop eating compulsively.

Your perception of yourself may be grossly inaccurate at times and it can change as your feelings about yourself change.

Part of stopping compulsive eating permanently is accepting each bodily change as a *natural* part of life.

Do not dress to look like or try to be someone else. *Be yourself* (everyone else is taken anyway). Be comfortable and breathe. Choose what suits you.

Make or revise your personal plan for taking the best possible care of your body—a plan designed by you and for you that exactly fits your special needs. Then promise yourself that you will follow it as often as possible. Remind yourself that you wouldn't break promises you make to other people. Vow to treat this promise to yourself equally seriously.

Look in the mirror. Tell yourself you could be bigger, you could be smaller and accept yourself as you are now. Self-acceptance and self-love *must* be primary in your life.

It is essential to know, and to believe, deep down in your adult heart of hearts, that you were not responsible for any abuse you suffered as a child. Children simply are not responsible. Adults are. *If anyone treated you with disrespect, if any adult hurt you in any way, shame on them. Be proud of yourself. You survived.*

You must feel a flow, a give and take, of loving energy in your life in order to thrive and to feel good about your relationships with others *and* with yourself.

For you to thrive in relationships, grow through them and not run to food when you feel threatened, you need to behave assertively, honestly, clearly and in an open-hearted way.

You can never rid yourself entirely of the negative voices within yourself. It is part of your humanness to have them. You can, however, learn ways to recognize those voices quickly, give yourself positive messages, break the self-destructive cycle, and resume control.

Black and white thinking stops the flow of your experience and leads you to a negative and self-destructive place. There are many shades of gray to be aware of in any situation. Open your mind and heart and take in the whole picture. You may discover many options that you were previously unaware of.

If you set perfection as your goal, you will be *forever* frustrated and your Chew will remain "in charge."

The messages you receive from society are clear: you are never all right just as you are. *Society is wrong.*

If you think all will be wonderful when you reach a certain goal, you will find when you get "there" there is no "there" there. There will always be more issues to work on, more goals to achieve. *Life is a process, not a conclusion.*

Where are you on your list of priorities? Are you even on the list? Put yourself there. You must *always* be number one.

There is no right or wrong way to develop your spiritual self and there is no way to do it perfectly either.

Spirituality is different and unique to each of us. It does, however, mean putting aside the distractions of your life temporarily and going inside to notice the feelings you are having and to listen to what your own voices are telling you. *That you acknowledge the spirit within yourself is what counts.*

It is necessary to nurture yourself. When was the last time you *really* paid attention to yourself?

The more focused you are on your outward appearance and the approval you do or don't receive from outside sources, the more difficult it is to journey within and hear your own voice.

Going inside to attend to yourself and your needs is an essential step in the process of letting go of *any* addiction.

You make a plan, revise it, revise it again. But you are always learning, always changing and always getting closer to yourself. *There are no mistakes, only lessons.*

Appreciating yourself is necessary if you are to treat yourself in a loving way.

Think of changing your compulsive eating behavior as an opportunity to make changes in many areas of your life. Think of your physical, emotional, societal and spiritual needs and then make alterations accordingly.

As you shed old negative beliefs about yourself, you will rediscover the sparkling, curious, precious little being that you *are* and *have always been.* Then you will be truly ready to nurture your body and your spirit.

Being sexual is natural. Sexuality is a beautiful, spiritual part of you and is to be celebrated—not hidden away under a blanket of anxiety, guilt and shame.

Even though it may seem awkward or scary at first, it is crucial to be true to yourself and to set boundaries that feel appropriate and safe for you. *If you do not, you will continue to eat your way through the confusing and painful feelings that you will experience.*

You will need to talk about your fears, your feelings and your progress with someone. *Trying to do it all by yourself is a set up for failure.* You must develop a good, strong support system and use it.

The more you develop a positive attitude and notice the humor in your life, the more calm and loving you will feel and the more gently you will treat yourself. The more gently you treat yourself, the less likely you will be to feel tense, to punish yourself by over-eating and the more tame your Chew will become.

No matter how you connect with others, the connecting itself is what's important. Connection validates you and empowers you to feel accepted, to grow and to change.

As long as you try to tailor your looks, your behaviors and your feelings to match the expectations of others, you will not feel good about yourself. You will continue taking care of yourself in the ways that you have in the past—self-destructively.

If you are to conquer your compulsive eating behaviors permanently and feel in control of your life, you must express yourself fully. There is great freedom in self-expression. With it comes a feeling of being alive and empowered. When you feel this way, stuffing yourself with food is not an option.

If you remain out of touch with your feelings and experiences in the present, you will continue the pattern of over-eating, beating yourself up emotionally for it and then eating even more. The past is gone and the future is not yet here to command your attention. Bring yourself back to the present. You need all of your energy to *be here now.*

When things seem the darkest, try to realize that there are life lessons hidden within each experience and that you are learning and growing all the time. You don't have to like the situation or the pain to work on accepting it as part of your life. When you are having a hard time, embrace your pain as useful and necessary for your development. The less you resist a painful situation the more quickly it will pass and the less likely you will be to eat your way through it.

You need quiet time. You need to breathe and to reflect. *You need to set aside time regularly to go within and to listen to your own voice.* Only then can you hear the words of wisdom that you have deep within your core self.

Making self-loving choices continuously may be your intention however actually doing so every time is impossible. It is possible, however, to make a majority of self-loving choices and that is the goal —*being perfect is not.*

Because life is so full of distractions, you must remind yourself again and again to make yourself top priority. You need to *nurture yourself often* and in as many ways as you can—physically, emotionally, socially, and spiritually.

When the urge to binge strikes, tell yourself you will make a choice to eat or not to eat only after you have thought it through and done at least one of the activities on your list (like reading this list of concepts, for example).

When you least feel like taking action—when you feel helpless, ashamed, frustrated, alone, unhappy, anxious, etc.—is the *most important* time to show yourself and your Chew that you are in control.

If you beat yourself up for past behavior, you will reinforce your negative self-concept and assure that you remain caught in a negative spin. Do as many positive things as you can to help your wheel move in a positive direction once again.

Do something *every day* to remind yourself that you are responsible for yourself and your choices and that you are a loving spirit. This practice will set you free from the prison of compulsive eating.

None of this will be effective without a sincere commitment on your part, and to make such a fervent commitment, you *must* love and nurture yourself.

Be gentle with yourself and, once again, remember, there really are *no mistakes, only lessons.*

Denise Lamothe is available to present lectures or workshops in your area. For further information regarding her services or to offer comments, feedback or suggestions:

You may contact her directly at:

Telephone/ FAX: (603) 679-2432

E-Mail: QUESTDCL@aol.com

PO Box 933, Epping, New Hampshire 03042

Don't forget to visit Denise Lamothe's website often at:

http://www.questover.com

To order additional copies of *The Taming of the Chew*, see the coupon at the end of this book.

Other Workshops by Denise Lamothe include:

Counseling—how to listen and help

Communicating Effectively—enhancing connections

Resolving Conflicts—in and out of the work place

Understanding Eating Disorders—understanding and helping ourselves and others

Managing Stress Creatively—developing good coping skills

Surviving Midlife and Menopause—what to expect and how to manage the changes

Living a Holistic Lifestyle—pausing to reflect and reevaluate

Coping with Death and Dying—understanding and growing from the experience

Learning and Growing through Transition—using the crisis of transition as opportunity

Growing through Divorce/Separation—accepting and moving on

Enhancing Self-Esteem—what self-esteem is and how to impact positively upon it

Nurturing our Creativity—making time for fun and creative personal growth

Making Crisis an Opportunity—yours and others'

Being Assertive—finding the balance point between non-assertion and aggression

Looking at Women's Psychology—understanding gender differences

Functioning Optimally in a Group Setting—as participant or facilitator

Understanding Homophobia—elimination through education

Creating Fulfilling Relationships—enhancing connections with others

Reading List

T HE books on this reading list have been chosen because each offers useful information to help you enhance your knowledge in any of the areas we have touched upon—physical, emotional, social and spiritual. Because many of these suggested readings cover topics related to more than one area, I have coded the books in this way:

> P= Physical
> E= Emotional
> So= Social
> Sp= Spiritual

P *Are You Confused?* Paavo Airola. Health Plus Publishers

P *Ayurvedic Healing: A Comprehensive Guide.* David Frawley. Morson Publishing

P *Fit for Life.* Harvey & Marilyn Diamond. Warner Books

P *Fit for Life II.* Harvey & Marilyn Diamond. Warner Books

P *Health and Healing.* Andrew Weil. Houghton Mifflin Co.

P *Healthy Healing—A Guide to Self-Healing for Everyone.* Linda Rector Page. Healthy Healing

P *Holistic Herbal.* David Hoffmann. Element Books

P *Juice Fasting.* Steve Meyerowitz. The Sprout House

P   *Low Fat Living*. Robert & Leslie Cooper. Rodale Press

P   *Natural Health, Natural Medicine*. Andrew Weil. Houghton Mifflin Co.

P   *New Choices in Natural Healing*. Bill Gottlieb, Editor-in-Chief. Rodale Press

P   *Outsmarting the Female Fat Cell*. Debra Waterhouse. Hyperion

P   *Prescription for Nutritional Healing*. James & Phyllis Balch. Avery Publishing Group Inc.

P   *Spontaneous Healing*. Andrew Weil. Ballantine Books

E   *Living, Loving and Learning*. Leo Buscaglia. Charles B. Slack, Inc.

So   *Toward a New Psychology of Women*. Jean Baker Miller. Beacon Press

So   *Fat is a Feminist Issue*. Susie Orbach. Paddington Press Ltd.

So   *Fat is a Feminist Issue II*. Susie Orbach. Berkley Publishing Corp.

Sp   *Emmanuel's Book*. Pat Rodegast & Judith Stanton. Bantam Books

Sp   *Emmanuel's Book II*. Pat Rodegast & Judith Stanton. Bantam Books

Sp   *Emmanuel's Book III*. Pat Rodegast & Judith Stanton. Bantam Books

P, E *For Yourself: The Fulfillment of Female Sexuality*. Lonnie Barbach. Doubleday and Co.

P, E   *Natural Alternatives to Prozac.* Michael Murray.
              William Morrow & Co.

P, E   *Nature's Prozac.* Judith Sachs. Prentice Hall

P, E   *The Natural Gormet.* Annemarie Colbin. Ballentine Books

P, E   *Why Weight? A Guide to Ending Compulsive Eating.*
              Geneen Roth. Penguin Books

P, So   *Diet for a New America.* John Robbins. Stillpoint
              Publishing

P, E, So   *Making Peace with Food.* Susan Kano. Harper and Row

P, E, So   *What to Do when Love Turns Violent.* Marian Betancourt.
              Harper Collins Publishers, Inc.

P, E, So   *Women's Bodies, Women's Wisdom.* Christiane Northrup.
              Bantam Books

P, E, Sp   *Ayurveda: A Life of Balance.* Maya Tiwari. Healing Arts
              Press

P, E, Sp   *Ayurvedic Cooking for Westerners.* Amadea Morningstar.
              Lotus Press

P, E, Sp   *Make the Connection: Ten Steps to a Better Body and a
              Better Life.* Bob Greene & Oprah Winfrey. Hyperion

P, E, Sp   *Perfect Weight.* Deepak Chopra. Crown Trade Paperbacks

P, E, Sp   *The American Holistic Health Association Complete Guide
              to Alternative Medicine.* William Collinge.
              Warner Books

P, E, Sp   *The Western Guide to Feng Shui.* Terah Kathryn Collins.
              Hay House

P, E, So, Sp   *Appetites.* Geneen Roth. (2 audio tapes). Sounds True

P, E, So, Sp   *One Bowl.* Don Gerrard. Random House

P, E, So, Sp   *Succulent Wild Woman: Dancing with your Wonder-full Self.* Sark. Simon and Shuster

P, E, So, Sp   *The Natural Remedy Book for Women.* Diane Stein. The Crossing Press

P, E, So, Sp   *Why People Don't Heal.* Caroline Myss. (2 audiotapes). Sounds True Audio

E, So   *Breaking Free from Compulsive Eating.* Geneen Roth. Signet

E, So   *In a Different Voice.* Carol Gilligan. Harvard University Press

E, So   *The Dance of Anger.* Harriet Goldhor Lerner. Harper and Row

E, So   *The New Assertive Woman.* Lynn Bloom, Karen Coburn & Joan Pearlman. Dell publishing

E, So   *When Women Stop Hating Their Bodies.* Jane Hirschmann & Carol Munter. Ballentine Books

E, So   *Women's Ways of Knowing.* Belenky, Clinchy, et al. Basic Books

E, Sp   *Being Peace.* Thich Nhat Hanh. Parallax Press

E, Sp   *Nourishing Wisdom.* Marc David. Harmony Books

E, Sp   *Peace Is Every Step.* Thich Nhat Hanh. Bantam Books

E, Sp   *The Language of Letting Go.* Melody Beattie. Hazelden Foundation

E, Sp   *The Miracle of Mindfulness.* Thich Nhat Hanh. Beacon
         Press

E, Sp   *The Road Less Traveled.* M. Scott Peck. Simon & Schuster

E, So, Sp   *Co-Dependant No More.* Melody Beattie. Hazelden
         Foundation

E, So, Sp   *Guilt is The Teacher, Love is the Lesson.* Joan Borysenko.
         Warner Books

E, So, Sp   *The Artist's Way.* Julia Cameron. G.P. Putnam's Sons

E, So, Sp   *When Food is Love: Exploring the Relationship between
         Eating and Intimacy.* Geneen Roth. Penguin Books

Resources

The American Holistic Health
  Association
AHHA – Dept C
PO Box 17400
Anaheim, CA 92817-7400
(714) 779-6152

Office of Alternative Medicine (NIH)
Box 8218
Silver Springs, MD 20904
www.altmed.od.nih.gov
(301) 495-4957

Office of Alternative Medicine (NIH)
9000 Rockville Pike, Mailstop 2182
Bldg. 31, Rm. 5B-38
Bethesda, MD 20892
(800) 531-1794

Am. Assoc. of Oriental Medicine
433 Front St.
Catasauqua, PA 18032
www.aaom.org
(610) 433-2448

Nat'l Cert. Comm for Acupuncture
  and Oriental Medicine
PO Box 97075
Washington, DC 20090
www.nccaom.org
(202) 232-1404

College of Maharishi
  Ayur-Veda Health Center
PO Box 282
Fairfield, IA 52556
www.theraj.com
(515) 472-5866

Am. Assn. Of Naturopathic
  Physicians
2366 Eastlake Ave
Suite 322
Seattle, WA 98102
(206) 323-7610

Am. Academy of Medical
  Acupuncture
5820 Wilshire Blvd.
Suite 500
Los Angeles, CA 90036
(800) 521-2262

Ayurvedic Institute
11311 Menaul NE, Suite A
Albuquerque NM 87112
www.ayurveda.com
(505) 291-9698

American Chiropractic Assn.
1701 Clarendon Blvd.
Arlington, VA 22209
www.americhiro.org
(703) 276-8800

American Massage Therapy Assn.
820 Davis St., Suite 100
Evanston, IL 60201
www.amtamassage.org
(708) 761-2682

Nurse Healers Professional Associates
1211 Locust St.
Philadelphia, PA 19107
(215) 545-8079

Herb Research Foundation
1007 Pearl St., Suite 200
Boulder, CO 80302
www.herbs.org
(303) 449-2265

Food and Drug Administration
5800 Fishers Lane
Rockville, MD 20857
www.vm.cfsan.fda.gov
(800) 332-0178
Med Watch: (800) 332-1088

Wilderness Transitions
(information about vision quests)
Wilderness Transitions
70 Rodeo Ave.
Sausalito, CA 94965
(415) 332-9558

The American Anorexia/Bulimia Assn.
AA/BA
165 West 46th Street, #1108
New York, NY 10036
(212) 575-6200

**International Assn. Of Yoga
Therapists**
20 Sunnyside Ave.
Suite A243
Mill Valley, CA 94941
(415) 866-1147

American Botanical Council
PO Box 1660
Austin, TX 78720
www.herbalgram.org
(512)331-8868

Canterbury Farms
16185 S.W. 108th Ave.
Tigard, Oregon
canfarms@spiritone.com
(503) 968-8269

American Herbalists Guild
PO Box 1683
Soquel, CA 95073

National Domestic Abuse
Hotline 1-800-799-SAFE

**National Eating Disorder
Organization**
NEDO
6655 South Yale Ave.
Tulsa, OK 74136
telephone (918) 481-4044
fax (918) 481-4076

The Center for Eating Disorders
c/o St. Joseph's Medical Center
7620 York Rd.
Towson, MD 21204
(410) 427-2100

Index

Further Reflections

Further Reflections

For further information about the many services offered
by Denise Lamothe,

you may contact her directly at:

PO Box 933, Epping, NH 03042

telephone/fax 603-679-2432

Email: QuestDCL@aol.com

. . . and don't forget to visit her website often at:

http://www.questover.com

To order more copies of

The Taming of the Chew
A Holistic Guide to Stopping Compulsive Eating

Please rush me _____ copy/copies of *The Taming of the Chew* by Denise Lamothe, Psy.D., H.H.D. I am enclosing $11.95 per copy plus $3.95 per copy postage and handling. I understand that if I am not completely satisfied with this book, I may return the undamaged copy by insured parcel post within ten days and receive a complete refund of my purchase price.

Name _____ Telephone _____

Address _____ City _____ State _____ Zip _____

CK __ MC __ VISA __ AM EX __ # _____ Expiration Date _____

Number of Copies _____ Total enclosed $ _____ Signature _____

☐ Check here if you would like your name added to Denise Lamothe's mailing list.

Please make checks payable to: Dr. Denise Lamothe
And mail to: Questover Books, P O Box 933, Epping, NH 03042